The Vertebrate Pigmentary System: From Pigment Cells to Disorders

Authored by

Sharique A. Ali

&

Naima Parveen

Department of Biotechnology and Zoology
Saifia College of Science
Barkatullah University, Bhopal
India

The Vertebrate Pigmentary System: From Pigment Cells to Disorders

Authors: Sharique A. Ali & Naima Parveen

ISBN (Online): 978-981-14-9158-0

ISBN (Print): 978-981-14-9156-6

ISBN (Paperback): 978-981-14-9157-3

need for a court order if at any point you breach any terms of this License Agreement. In no event will any delay or failure by Bentham Science Publishers in enforcing your compliance with this License Agreement constitute a waiver of any of its rights.

3. You acknowledge that you have read this License Agreement, and agree to be bound by its terms and conditions. To the extent that any other terms and conditions presented on any website of Bentham Science Publishers conflict with, or are inconsistent with, the terms and conditions set out in this License Agreement, you acknowledge that the terms and conditions set out in this License Agreement shall prevail.

Bentham Science Publishers Pte. Ltd.
80 Robinson Road #02-00
Singapore 068898
Singapore
Email: subscriptions@benthamscience.net

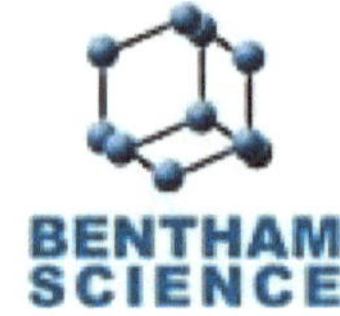

CONTENTS

PREFACE

Although various vertebrate classes, from fishes to mammals are each distinctive but they possess many common features from phylogenetic point of view, making it important to understand their comparative biology. One general feature that has long commanded scientific attention is the integumental pigmentary system. Due to this, one can see the butterflies, fishes and birds with striking colors, along with the human beings showing different skin tones. This is due to the presence of a chemically inert and stable pigment known as melanin which is formed inside the melanosomes within the melanophores or melanocytes. Alteration in any structure and function of the pigmentary cells in mammals including human beings, affects the process of melanogenesis, which may lead to pigmentary disorders including hyperpigmentation or hypopigmentation. Vitiligo, albinism, post inflammatory hyperpigmentation, melasma, solar lentigos are some of the diseases of hypo and hyperpigmentation. Although many pigmentary disorders are mainly of cosmetic concern, the condition may be devastating and stigmatizing and can have a negative psychosocial impact on human life, requiring the clinician to be sensitive to the overall impact of the disorder and treat it accordingly.

Despite various treatment strategies, including noncytotoxic laser, topical formulations, chemical peeling and skin grafting practiced by dermatologists and cosmetologists, the impact of pigmentary disorders remains dreadful. In contrast to this, we have found significant advancement in this field of research using herbal products, demonstrating the growing interest of academic researchers and pharmaceutical companies in developing successful natural agents and their formulations for the treatment of pigmentary disorders.

In this book, '*The Vertebrate Pigmentary System: From pigment cells to Disorders*', we intend to provide fundamental knowledge of the structural and functional aspects of vertebrate pigment cells from their origin to different stages of development along with their specific regulating receptors and markers. Signalling pathways of skin melanocytes along with the diseases in human beings associated with their disruption, have been discussed in detail. Concurrently, the etiologies of pigmentary disorders and the various therapeutic approaches for their treatment are the important chapters of the book with recent and updated information. Interestingly, the part of the book including potentials of natural products based treatment for hypo and hyperpigmentation will definitely captivate the readers to have interesting reads.

The outcome of the research is based on several decades of research in pigment cell biology in our laboratory. The book is exceptional from previously published volumes on different aspects of pigment cell biology as it contains updated information from the basics of pigment cells to the structure and function of normal cells and their consequent abnormalities with treatment options in a single volume. Hence, it is ideally suited as a basic guide for newcomers in the field of pigment cell biology, and a handy source of information for academicians as well as for practitioners in medical and industrial backgrounds.

We hope that the readers involved in research on pigment cells and their related disorders will find the chapters of the book valuable and inspiring so that they may elicit further research in pigment cells, pigmentary disorders and their treatment with natural plant based ingredients.

We wish to acknowledge the work of those at Bentham Science Publishers who patiently coordinated the production of this book. We are especially grateful for the timely efforts made by Ms. Salma Sarfraz (Senior Publication Manager, Bentham Science Publishers, UAE) to bring out this academic venture. Finally, we gratefully acknowledge our families and friends who, throughout this period, provided strong support, despite having to put up with our frequent absences and distractions.

CONSENT FOR PUBLICATION

Not applicable

CONFLICT OF INTEREST

The authors declare no conflict of interest, financial or otherwise.

ACKNOWLEDGEMENTS

Declared none.

Sharique A. Ali
&
Naima Parveen
Saifia College of Science
Barkatullah University, Bhopal
India

CHAPTER 1

Origin, Proliferation and Development of Vertebrate Pigment Cells-Melanophores and Melanocytes

Abstract: Skin color in vertebrates predominantly depends on the presence of specialized cells that produce pigment. These special cells absorb or reflect light in a specific way to impart color to the skin and are called as chromatophores. Chromatophores are grouped into melanophores, erythrophores, xanthophores, leucophores and iridophores which largely depend on the pigment they produce. Melanophores are the most important type of chromatophores responsible for dorsal pigmentation in many vertebrates including fishes, amphibians and reptiles. In birds and mammals, melanophores are called melanocytes. All melanophores or melanocytes store thousands of dark brown/black biopolymer pigment melanins, packaged into membrane bound intra-cytoplasmic vesicles called as melanosomes. Melanophores or melanocytes originated from the neural crest cells, induced by several extracellular signals. Melanoblasts, precursor of melanocytes migrate, proliferate, differentiate and spread to their final destination in the basal layer of epidermis and hair follicles, however, distribution of melanocytes varies among different species. The embryonic development of melanocytes offers an opportunity to better understand the concept of vertebrate pigmentation. Thus the present chapter provides siginificant knowledge on the vertebrate pigment cells from origin to different stages of their development.

Keywords: Chromatophores, Epidermis, Melanoblast, Melanocytes, Melanophores, Neural crest cells.

1. INTRODUCTION

The various colour changes that many animals undergo are remarkably brought about by the pigment cells present in their skin and scales. The colour bearing cells are known as "chromatophores" originated from Greek word *khrōma* meaning 'color' and *phoros* meaning 'bearing'. Chromatophores are the pigment containing and light reflection cells found in fishes, amphibians and reptiles. Chromatophores are classified into different groups depending on what pigment they produce. Among them, those impart their characteristic color by absorbing light are melanophores, erythrophores and xanthophores, whereas those that reflect light are leucophores and iridophores [1 - 4].

Sharique A. Ali & Naima Parveen

Melanophores are brown black, xanthophores are yellow, erythrophores are red while leucophores and iridophores are white and reflecting. Melanophores are the most common type of chromatophores and are responsible for most of the dorsal pigmentation in all vertebrates including fishes, amphibians and reptiles [5]. Melanophores can be further divided into two types on the basis of their location and appearance: dermal melanophores and epidermal melanophores. Dermal melanophores are the flat cells with processes that radiate upward and outwards from the main body of the cells. These types of cells are responsible for rapid, chromomotor color change in cold blooded vertebrates [6]. Epidermal melanophores are present in dermo-epidermal junction having long thin dendritic processes and spread among the neighbouring keratinocytes. This arrangement allows the melanosomes to get transferred to dermal keratinocytes and in birds and mammals it is this deposition of melanin that decides the pigmentation of their skin and hair. These types of cells are not involved in rapid chromomotor colour change and due to their limited capability to move their pigment they are called as melanocytes [7].

Melanocytes in mammals produce two types of melanin: the brown or black eumelanin and the yellow or red pheomelanin. Lower vertebrates do not synthesize pheomelanin [7]. Apart from integument, melanocytes are also found in the eye, the inner ear, and in a variety of other inner organs like the lung, the heart and the aorta [6]. A variety of histological observations were brought to understand the origin of pigment cells, melanophores or melanocytes. But then, it has clearly been established that melanophores are originated from the neural crest cells (NCC) through many developmental stages, regulated by various proteins [8]. Neural crest cells are the embryonic population of cells which are formed at the border between neural plate and the neighbouring surface ectoderm. At the early stages of development, the precursor of melanophores, melanoblasts cannot be differentiated from other embryonic cells as they are at first without pigment. But after differentiation, proliferation, migration, they finally reach their destination in the skin. In the present chapter, an attempt has been made to explain the origin of melanophores at various stages of development in different vertebrates including fishes, amphibians, reptiles, birds and mammals.

2. ORIGIN OF MELANOPHORES/MELANOCYTES

To facilitate the understanding of the relationship of the factors, genetic or environmental, that is essentially involved in the development of a system of pigmentation, it is extremely important to know the source of the pigmentary unit, the melanophore or the melanocyte. A wide variety of histological observations on embryonic and adult tissues of nearly all classes of vertebrates has been brought to bear upon the problem of origin of melanophore [9]. But now, it is clearly established that neural crest (NC) is the source of all pigment cells in fishes, amphibians, reptiles, birds and mammals. In the early stages of development, the pigment cells cannot be distinguished morphologically from other embryonic cells. They are at first without pigment and due to this their true origin cannot be ascertained easily. But with the introduction and perfection of precise techniques it became possible to analyze the inherent development of embryonic tissues [10].

Melanophores are derived from pluripotent neural crest cells (NCC) which are the transient group of cells derived from the dorsal aspect of neural tube during vertebrate embryonic development. They are multipotent, long range migratory embryo, and have a capacity to develop a number of differentiated cell types. Due to these reasons, neural crest is also known as fourth embryonic layer. In addition to the development of melanophores, they give rise to adrenal medulla, glial cells, cardiac cells, neurons, and craniofacial tissues [11]. Neural crest cells are grouped into four regionally distributed populations: cranial, vagal, trunk and sacral. Melanocytes have largely originated from cranial and trunk located NCC. In human beings, melanocytes residing in the skin of the head; originated from the cranial NCC where as the melanocytes of the remaining parts of the body came from the trunk NCC [12].

Originating from the border between the dorsal neural tube and overlying ectoderm, neural crest cells come out following closure of the neural tube during neurulation. During initiation, NC population needs the action of various transcription factors such as Msx1, Sox10, Pax3, FoxD3, Snail2, AP-2, Zic1, microphthalmia induced transcription factor (MITF), endothelin 3 and endothelin receptor B (EDNRB) [13, 14]. The expression of these factors is regulated by Wnt and bone morphogenic protein (BMP) signaling [15]. These proteins or transcription factors along with the signaling pathways give integrated spatial and temporal signals to create the proper environment for development and migration [16, 17].

Neural crest cells migrate widely around the embryo, during which they differentiate into specialized cell types. The providence of NCC depends on several environmental factors they meet on the migratory pathways. At the trunk, from somite eight to twenty eight, NCC emerge after an epitheliomesenchymal transition (EMT), proliferate comprehensively and follow two main migration paths; the dorso-lateral and the dorso-ventral pathways. The cells which migrate along the dorso-lateral pathway, between somite and ectoderm, are considered as the main source for melanocytes whereas the cells that migrate dorso-ventrally are thought to produce peripheral nervous system and adrenal medulla [12, 18]. But, there is an evidence of the fact that a fraction of melanocytes arise from cells migrating first ventrally and then along the nerves. Schwann cells (present in nerve sheath) also have the potential to produce melanocytes. Schwann cells when cultured *in vitro*, dedifferentiate into glial melanocytic progenitor that give rise to melanocytes. Hence, ventrally migrating cells either differentiate into neurons or maintained as multipotent cells which differentiate into the cells forming myelin sheath or melanocytes [19, 20]. Flow diagram of melanocytes development from neural crest cells (NCC) is shown in Fig. (**1**).

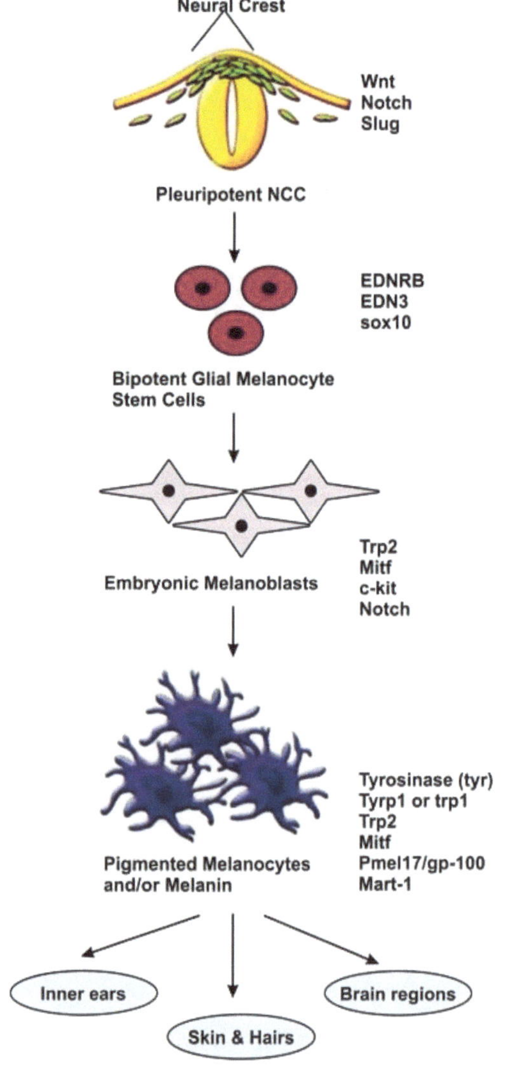

Fig. (1). Development of melanocytes from neural crest cells (NCC).

The findings of Cramer and Fesyuk [21] strongly supported the hypothesis that melanocyte precursors originated from dermis cells, they have demonstrated that prenatal nevi begin as intradermal nevi. It has also been suggested that development of prenatal nevi may be from the precursors of Schwann cells that appear near epidermis along cutaneous nerve, may respond to factors secreted by epidermal cells and differentiate into melanocytes. Cutaneous nerves grow from the deep dermis near the epidermis and they branch and form a neurocutaneous unit. Precursors for melanocytes migrate to the epidermis and prenatal nevi may develop consequently. The investigation that epidermal melanocytes molecularly differ from dermal melanocytes seems to support assumption about double origin of skin melanocytes [22]. Hence, skin melanocytes either develop directly from NCC populating the skin through dorsolateral migratory pathway or are derived from ventrally migrating precursors forming the myelin around the cutaneous nerves [23].

3. STUDIES IN SUPPORT OF NEURAL CREST ORIGIN OF MELANOPHORES IN DIFFERENT CLASSES OF VERTEBRATES

Amphibians are the first group of vertebrates in which information was obtained for origin of pigment cells from neural crest. A study conducted by Harrison [24], on the growth of nerve fibres in tissue cultures showed that pigmented cells formed from pieces of medullary cord. He thought they had their origin from the ganglion crest. Holtfreter [25] strongly supported the neural crest origin theory of pigment cells. He found evidences from their various transplantation experiments done on *Triton* embryo. DuShane [26] while working with *Amblystoma*, came across that if the neural folds (primordial of the neural crest) was removed in the neurula stage resulted in an entire loss of pigment cells in the operated (trunk) region; and when the separated folds were grown in culture medium or transplanted to the ventral region of other embryo, they produced several pigment cells. At tail-bud stages, after closure of the neural folds, the extirpated crest region transplanted heteroplastically between two pigmented embryos consistently produced pigment cells of the donor type.

Similarly, Twitty [27], Twitty and Bodenstein [28] and Raven [29] confirmed the neural crest origin of pigment cells while working with several species of *Triturus*. The study was extended by Bytinsky-Salz [30] through xenoplastic transplantation experiment done on anurans. He has found that all types of pigment cells; guanophore or melanophores were arising from the neural crest of the head and trunk region. Additionally, while working with amphibian eye; Barden [31] investigated that xanthophore, guanophore and melanophores found in iris and chorioidea originated from neural crest. Rosin [32] and Stearner [33] have elucidated the neural crest origin of melanophores found in epidermis. Stearner [33] have further shown that these types of melanophores are the sole source of dermal pigmentation in adults of various species. At present, a huge body of literature is available showing that all types of pigment cells; xanthophores, guanophores and melanophores that develop in various parts of amphibians are originated from neural crest [34 - 36].

In birds, there are several experiments pertaining to neural crest origin of melanophores. An interesting experiment conducted by Dorris [37] has shown that culture of neural crest of the pre-otic region of early chick embryos of various breeds produced melanophores. By means of culture of intracoelomic and other grafts from various axial levels of embryos of different varieties fowl and other birds, Ris [38] was able to correlate the presence of pigment cells in the grafts with the morphological development of neural crest at the time of isolation. He has concluded that only those isolates known to contain neural crest are capable of producing melanophores in grafts. The origin of the retinal and chorioidal pigments of the eye in fowl was also demonstrated by Ris [38]. The retinal pigment arises *in situ,* they do not occur in branched cells. However, the pigment of the iris and chorioides produced in branched cells, melanophores which were identical with those in skin and mesoderm and were also derived from neural crest. It was mentioned that the other pigment cells found in amphibians such as xanthophores, and guanophores do not exist in birds. The most widely occurring lipochrome pigments found within the feather cells of birds are not derived from the specialized migratory pigment forming cells. They are dissolved in the fat droplets deposited in cells of barb ridges prior to the onset of keratinization [39, 40].

The mammalian embryo in which the origin of melanophores from the neural crest has been demonstrated for the first time is the mouse embryo. Similar experiments were performed as that was used for describing the origin of melanophores in birds. It involves the isolation of tissues at different developmental stages from various axial levels and their successive transplantation to the embryonic coelom of White Leghorn chick hosts. The results of a series of experiments with embryos of a homozygous black strain of mouse have been demonstrated that those tissues having cells migrating from neural crest, presumptive neural crest, or histologically recognizable neural crest, can only produce melanophores [41, 42].

Subsequently, there has been little attention received for the origin of melanophores in remaining vertebrate groups, the fishes and the reptiles. It is extremely probable that melanophore origin in fishes and reptiles is also linked with neural crest differentiation. It was evident from the transplantation experiment of Lopashov [43] on teleost embryos that the melanophores got derived from the anlage of the central nervous system. Other researchers also gave some clues on the neural crest origin of melanophores [8, 44, 45]. Dooley *et al.* [46], working with zebra fish, demonstrated that during embryogenesis larval melanophores developed directly from neural crest cells migrating along dorsolateral and ventromedial paths. But, the embryonic origin of the melanophores comes out during juvenile development in the integument to contribute to the striking color of the fishes, remain intangible.

4. MIGRATION OF MELANOPHORES

It has been demonstrated clearly that melanophores originated from neural crest cells but the question next arises as to how and when they reach those parts of the body in which they are later found and at what stage NC gets features of melanoblast, a precursor to melanophores/melanocytes. But, the results of the different experiments conducted were not able to find out the answer of the question and the exact pathway for melanoblast migration is not known so far. Pigment cells are capable of independent movement but much of their migratory activity depends upon their contact with other tissues. Adhesion molecules such as cadherins, integrins, and extracellular matrix are possibly involved in it [47, 48].

Cadherins, a family of glycoproteins is involved in calcium dependent cell adhesion, cytoskeleton regulation and cell signaling. During development melanoblasts express distinct cadherins. Neural crest cells while delaminate from the epithelium, they express cadherin 6 and low levels of N-Cadherin. E- and P-cadherins are inadequately upregulated in migratory melanoblasts but neither is expressed on being arrived in the dermis. When the cells enter the epidermis, E-cadherins increase by 200 folds and interact with E-cadherin expressing keratinocytes. However, E-cadherins are downregulated again when melanoblasts enter hair follicles and exclusively express P-cadherin. The melanocytes remain in epidermis continue to express E-cadherin while those in the dermis express N-cadherin [49, 50]. Some workers have studied the involvement of another protein β –integrin in melanoblast migration. β – integrin is a member of a transmembrane protein family that serves as major binding partners for extracellular matrix components. But their relevance in migration of melanoblasts remains unclear. On the whole, the cell migration regulation involves a variety of protein molecules that all collaborate to ensure whether the cells travel on the right track or in the correct location [51, 52].

After cell specification melanoblasts proliferate and reach their final destinations in the epidermis and hair follicles. It takes place at 6-8 weeks and by 12-13 weeks, many of the melanoblasts gets localized in the epidermis. It remains indefinite that the stream of melanoblasts to the epidermis is controlled [53]. Some investigations have showed that melanoblasts could stay in the dermis. Dermal melanocytes were observed during human fetal development. While travelling to their destinations, melanoblasts successively express melanogenic genes, most of them are regulated by MITF. MITF stimulates the expression of anti apoptotic genes Bcl2 and Hif-1α. It also stimulates the transcription of the gene encoding cyclin dependent kinase-2 (CDK2) that promotes the G-S transition during the cell cycle and hence promotes cell proliferation. MITF also stimulates TBX2, a transcription factor that represses the p21 expression which is a protein inducing growth arrest. Despite of promoting cell proliferation, MITF also seems to be anti proliferative. That means it has both positive and negative effect on melanoblast proliferation. The appearance of tyrosinase which is the key enzyme for melanin synthesis is the indication of melanocyte maturation. Melanocytes ultimately inhabit in the skin and hair follicles, the oral mucosa, the iris, the choroid of the eye, meninges and inner ear [54 - 56]. The development and maturation of melanosomes is diagrammatically shown in Fig. (2).

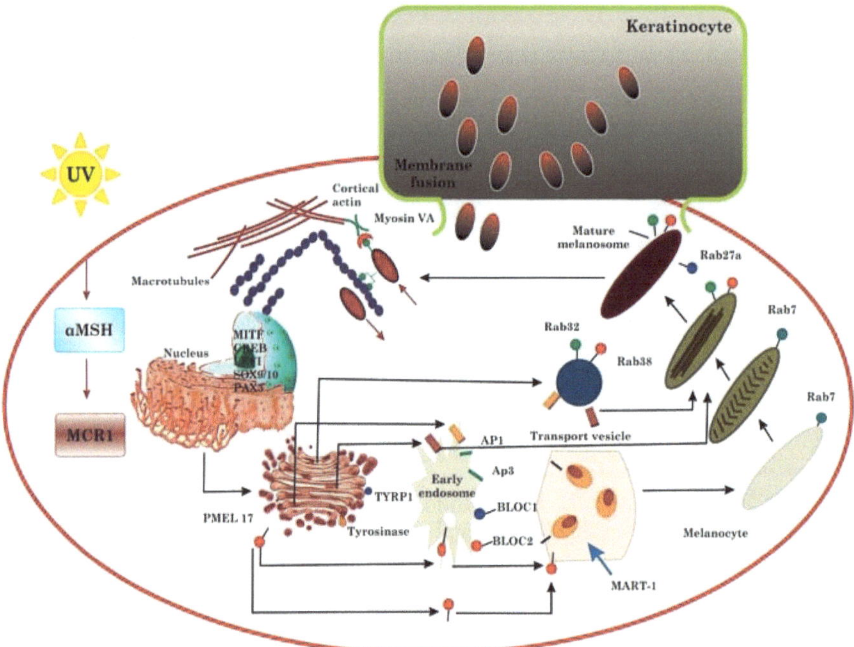

Fig. (2). Development and maturation of melanosomes.

5. MITF AS A CORE ELEMENT IN MELANOBLAST DIFFERENTIATION

In skin, melanoblast differentiation is characterized by melanisation and appearance of dendritic phenotype, and it depends a lot on MITF. Many of the genes involved in melanogenesis including *Dct*, tyrosinase, tyrosinase- related protein- 1 are the targets of MITF. The promoters of these genes contain a common *cis* element which is so-called M-box having Ephrussi (E) box in its core with the sequence 5'CATGTG3. E-boxes are predominantly present in genome and bound by an extensive array of basic-helix-loo-helix, basic-leucine-zipper, and basic-helix-loop-helix-leucine zipper transcription factors. Though flanking sequences affect the efficiency with which a specific factor bind to a particular E-Box, they are inadequate to elucidate the restriction of melanogenic genes to the melanocyte lineage [57, 58].

Furthermore, the combination of many distinct transcription factors and their post translational modifications is essential for this regulation. Post translational modifications such as phosphorylation and acetylation regulate the activity of MITF. Small ubiquitin like modifier (SUMO) side chains which are proteins of about 100 residues are capable of modifying MITF by attaching themselves to lysine of MITF. This modification reduces activity of MITF. Moreover, many studies have showed that some melanogenic genes are directly stimulated by a regulator of MITF *i.e.* SOX10. MITF also modulates cell shape by regulating the genes which are involved in dynamics of the actin cytoskeleton [59 - 62].

CONCLUSION

In lower vertebrates, a class of cells for coloration is known as melanophores and in higher vertebrates including birds and human beings, it is known as melanocytes. Melanophores or melanocytes are the flat and large cells, which possess several pigment granules; membrane bound organelles called melanosomes that contain melanin, a dark brown or black pigment. It is important to know the source of pigment cells, in order to understand the various factors involved in the development of a vertebrate pigmentary system. Many histological observations on embryonic and adult tissues of almost all pigment cells have been brought and some researchers are still continued to work to explain the origin of melanophores. Neural crest cells were found to be the source of all pigment cells in fishes, amphibians, reptiles, birds and mammals. Various regulatory genes and proteins are involved during the process of origin, development and differentiation of melanophores.

REFERENCES

[1]   Bagnara, J.T. Cytology and cytophysiology of non-melanophore pigment cells. *Int. Rev. Cytol.,* **1966**, *20*, 173-205.
[http://dx.doi.org/10.1016/S0074-7696(08)60801-3] [PMID: 5337298]

[2]   Fujii, R. *Chromatophores and pigments,* 3ʳᵈ ed; Academic Press: New York, **1969**, pp. 307-353.

[3]   Gopta, O.A.; Bloch, D.A.; Cherepanov, D.A.; Mulkidjanian, A.Y. Temperature dependence of the electrogenic reaction in the QB site of the *Rhodobacter sphaeroides* photosynthetic reaction center: the QA-QB --> QAQB- transition. *FEBS Lett.,* **1997**, *412*(3), 490-494.
[http://dx.doi.org/10.1016/S0014-5793(97)00842-9] [PMID: 9276452]

[4]   Míguez, D.G.; Muñuzuri, A.P. On the orientation of stripes in fish skin patterning. *Biophys. Chem.,* **2006**, *124*(2), 161-167.
[http://dx.doi.org/10.1016/j.bpc.2006.06.014] [PMID: 16844282]

[5]   Obika, M. Morphology of chromatophores of the medaka. *The fish biology journal Medaka.,* **1996**, *8*, 21-27.

[6]   Szydłowski, P.; Madej, J.P.; Mazurkiewicz-Kania, M. Histology and ultrastructure of the integumental chromatophores in tokay gecko (*Gekko gecko*) (Linnaeus, 1758) skin. *Zoomorphology,* **2017**, *136*(2), 233-240.
[http://dx.doi.org/10.1007/s00435-017-0348-9] [PMID: 28553007]

[7]   Aspengren, S.; Hedberg, D.; Sköld, H.N.; Wallin, M. New insights into melanosome transport in vertebrate pigment cells. *Int. Rev. Cell Mol. Biol.,* **2009**, *272*, 245-302.
[http://dx.doi.org/10.1016/S1937-6448(08)01606-7] [PMID: 19121820]

[8]   Quigley, I.K.; Turner, J.M.; Nuckels, R.J.; Manuel, J.L.; Budi, E.H.; MacDonald, E.L.; Parichy, D.M. Pigment pattern evolution by differential deployment of neural crest and post-embryonic melanophore lineages in Danio fishes. *Development,* **2004**, *131*(24), 6053-6069.
[http://dx.doi.org/10.1242/dev.01526] [PMID: 15537688]

[9]   Le Douarin, N. A biological cell labeling technique and its use in expermental embryology. *Dev. Biol.,* **1973**, *30*(1), 217-222.
[http://dx.doi.org/10.1016/0012-1606(73)90061-4] [PMID: 4121410]

[10]   Huang, X.; Saint-Jeannet, J.P. Induction of the neural crest and the opportunities of life on the edge. *Dev. Biol.,* **2004**, *275*(1), 1-11.
[http://dx.doi.org/10.1016/j.ydbio.2004.07.033] [PMID: 15464568]

[11]   Le Douarin, N.M.; Kalcheim, C. *The neural crest,* 2ⁿᵈ ed; Cambridge University Press: Cambridge, **1999**.
[http://dx.doi.org/10.1017/CBO9780511897948]

[12]   Le Douarin, N.M.; Creuzet, S.; Couly, G.; Dupin, E. Neural crest cell plasticity and its limits. *Development,* **2004**, *131*(19), 4637-4650.
[http://dx.doi.org/10.1242/dev.01350] [PMID: 15358668]

[13]   Steventon, B.; Carmona-Fontaine, C.; Mayor, R. Genetic network during neural crest induction: from cell specification to cell survival. *Semin. Cell Dev. Biol.,* **2005**, *16*(6), 647-654.
[http://dx.doi.org/10.1016/j.semcdb.2005.06.001] [PMID: 16084743]

[14]   Tobin, D.J. Aging of the hair follicle pigmentation system. *Int. J. Trichology,* **2009**, *1*(2), 83-93.
[http://dx.doi.org/10.4103/0974-7753.58550] [PMID: 20927229]

[15]   Abu-Elmagd, M.; Garcia-Morales, C.; Wheeler, G.N. Frizzled7 mediates canonical Wnt signaling in neural crest induction. *Dev. Biol.,* **2006**, *298*(1), 285-298.
[http://dx.doi.org/10.1016/j.ydbio.2006.06.037] [PMID: 16928367]

[16]   Theveneau, E.; Mayor, R. Neural crest delamination and migration: from epithelium-to-mesenchyme transition to collective cell migration. *Dev. Biol.,* **2012**, *366*(1), 34-54.

[http://dx.doi.org/10.1016/j.ydbio.2011.12.041] [PMID: 22261150]

[17]   Milet, C.; Monsoro-Burq, A.H. Neural crest induction at the neural plate border in vertebrates. *Dev Biol.,* **2012**, *366*(1), 22-33 5.
[http://dx.doi.org/10.1016/j.ydbio.2012.01.013]

[18]   Dupin, E.; Real, C.; Glavieux-Pardanaud, C.; Vaigot, P.; Le Douarin, N.M. Reversal of developmental restrictions in neural crest lineages: transition from Schwann cells to glial-melanocytic precursors *in vitro. Proc. Natl. Acad. Sci. USA,* **2003**, *100*(9), 5229-5233.
[http://dx.doi.org/10.1073/pnas.0831229100] [PMID: 12702775]

[19]   Prasad, M.S.; Charney, R.M.; García-Castro, M.I. Specification and formation of the neural crest: Perspectives on lineage segregation. *Genesis,* **2019**, *57*(1), e23276.
[http://dx.doi.org/10.1002/dvg.23276] [PMID: 30576078]

[20]   Cramer, S.F.; Fesyuk, A. On the development of neurocutaneous units--implications for the histogenesis of congenital, acquired, and dysplastic nevi. *Am. J. Dermatopathol.,* **2012**, *34*(1), 60-81.
[http://dx.doi.org/10.1097/DAD.0b013e31822d071a] [PMID: 22197860]

[21]   Aoki, H.; Yamada, Y.; Hara, A.; Kunisada, T. Two distinct types of mouse melanocyte: differential signaling requirement for the maintenance of non-cutaneous and dermal *versus* epidermal melanocytes. *Development,* **2009**, *136*(15), 2511-2521.
[http://dx.doi.org/10.1242/dev.037168] [PMID: 19553284]

[22]   Sommer, L. Generation of melanocytes from neural crest cells. *Pigment Cell Melanoma Res.,* **2011**, *24*(3), 411-421.
[http://dx.doi.org/10.1111/j.1755-148X.2011.00834.x] [PMID: 21310010]

[23]   Harrison, R.G. The outgrowth of the nerve fiber as a mode of protoplasmic movement. *J. Exp. Zool.,* **1910**, *9*(4), 787-846.
[http://dx.doi.org/10.1002/jez.1400090405] [PMID: 13711840]

[24]   Holtfreter, J. About the Rearing of Isolated Parts of the Amphibian Germ: I. Method of Tissue Culture *in vivo. Wilhelm Roux Arch. Entwickl. Mech. Org.,* **1929**, *117*, 421-510.
[http://dx.doi.org/10.1007/BF02110971] [PMID: 28354659]

[25]   Dushane, G.P. An experimental study of the origin of pigment cells in Amphibia. *J. Exp. Zool.,* **1935**, *72*, 1.
[http://dx.doi.org/10.1002/jez.1400720102]

[26]   Twitty, V.C. Correlated genetic and embryological experiments in Triturus: I and II. *J. Exp. Zool.,* **1936**, *74*, 239-302.
[http://dx.doi.org/10.1002/jez.1400740206]

[27]   Twitty, V.C.; Bodenstein, D. Correlated genetic and embryological experiments on Triturus. *J. Exp. Zool.,* **1939**, *81*, 357-398.
[http://dx.doi.org/10.1002/jez.1400810304]

[28]   Raven, C.P. To the development of the Ganglienleiste V: About the differentiation of the trunk ganglia material. *Arch. Entwicklungsmech. Org.,* **1936**, *134*, 122-145.
[http://dx.doi.org/10.1007/BF00573467]

[29]   Bytinsky-Salz, H. Chromatophore studies II. Structure and determination of the adepidermal melanophoretic network at *Bombina. Arch. exptl. Zellforsch. Gewebeziicht,* **1938**, *22*, 132-170.

[30]   Thomas, A.J.; Erickson, C.A. The making of a melanocyte: the specification of melanoblasts from the neural crest. *Pigment Cell Melanoma Res.,* **2008**, *21*(6), 598-610.
[http://dx.doi.org/10.1111/j.1755-148X.2008.00506.x] [PMID: 19067969]

[31]   Barden, R.B. The origin and development of the chromatophores of the amphibian eye. *J. Exp. Zool.,* **1942**, *90*, 479-519.
[http://dx.doi.org/10.1002/jez.1400900309]

[32] Rosin, S. Experiments on the developmental physiology of pigmentation in amphibians. *Rev. Swiss. Zool,* **1943**, *50*, 485-578.

[33] Stearner, S.P. Pigmentation studies in salamanders, with especial reference to the changes at metamorphosis. *Physiol. Zool.,* **1946**, *19*(4), 375-404.
[http://dx.doi.org/10.1086/physzool.19.4.30151927] [PMID: 20285937]

[34] Bagnara, J.T.; Frost, S.K.; Matsumoto, J. On the development of pigment patterns in amphibians. *Am. Zool.,* **1978**, *18*, 301-312.
[http://dx.doi.org/10.1093/icb/18.2.301]

[35] Epperlein, H.H.; Löfberg, J. The development of the neural crest in amphibians. *Ann. Anat.,* **1993**, *175*(6), 483-499.
[http://dx.doi.org/10.1016/S0940-9602(11)80207-4] [PMID: 8297037]

[36] Eom, D.S.; Bain, E.J.; Patterson, L.B.; Grout, M.E.; Parichy, D.M. Long-distance communication by specialized cellular projections during pigment pattern development and evolution. *eLife,* **2015**, *4*, e12401.
[http://dx.doi.org/10.7554/eLife.12401] [PMID: 26701906]

[37] Dorris, F. The production of pigment *in vitro* by chick neural crest. *Wilhelm Roux Arch. Entwickl. Mech. Org.,* **1938**, *138*(3-4), 323-334.
[http://dx.doi.org/10.1007/BF00573807] [PMID: 28354525]

[38] Ris, H. An experimental study on the origin of melanophorescin birds. *Physiol. Zool.,* **1941**, *1941*(14), 48-66.
[http://dx.doi.org/10.1086/physzool.14.1.30151597]

[39] Desselberger, H.J. About the lipochrome of bird feather. *J. Ornithol.,* **1930**, *78*, 328-376.
[http://dx.doi.org/10.1007/BF01953327]

[40] Volker, O. The material basis of pigmentation of the birds. *Biol. Zentralbl.,* **1944**, *84*, 184.

[41] Rawles, M.E. The development of melanophores from embryonic mouse tissues grown in the coelom of chick embryos. *Proc. Natl. Acad. Sci. USA,* **1940**, *26*(12), 673-680.
[http://dx.doi.org/10.1073/pnas.26.12.673] [PMID: 16588410]

[42] Rawles, M.E. Origin of pigment cells from the neural crest in the mouse embryo. *Physiol. Zool.,* **1947**, *20*(3), 248-266.
[http://dx.doi.org/10.1086/physzool.20.3.30151958] [PMID: 20256541]

[43] Lopashov, G.V. Origins of pigment cells and visceral cartilage in teleosts. *C.R. Acad. Sci.USSR,* **1944**, *44*, 169-172.

[44] Quigley, I.K.; Manuel, J.L.; Roberts, R.A.; Nuckels, R.J.; Herrington, E.R.; MacDonald, E.L.; Parichy, D.M. Evolutionary diversification of pigment pattern in Danio fishes: differential fms dependence and stripe loss in D. albolineatus. *Development,* **2005**, *132*(1), 89-104.
[http://dx.doi.org/10.1242/dev.01547] [PMID: 15563521]

[45] Budi, E.H.; Patterson, L.B.; Parichy, D.M. Embryonic requirements for ErbB signaling in neural crest development and adult pigment pattern formation. *Development,* **2008**, *135*(15), 2603-2614.
[http://dx.doi.org/10.1242/dev.019299] [PMID: 18508863]

[46] Dooley, C.M.; Mongera, A.; Walderich, B.; Nüsslein-Volhard, C. On the embryonic origin of adult melanophores: the role of ErbB and Kit signalling in establishing melanophore stem cells in zebrafish. *Development,* **2013**, *140*(5), 1003-1013.
[http://dx.doi.org/10.1242/dev.087007] [PMID: 23364329]

[47] Ernfors, P. Cellular origin and developmental mechanisms during the formation of skin melanocytes. *Exp. Cell Res.,* **2010**, *316*(8), 1397-1407.
[http://dx.doi.org/10.1016/j.yexcr.2010.02.042] [PMID: 20211169]

[48] Larue, L.; de Vuyst, F.; Delmas, V. Modeling melanoblast development. *Cell. Mol. Life Sci.,* **2013**,

70(6), 1067-1079.
[http://dx.doi.org/10.1007/s00018-012-1112-4] [PMID: 22915137]

[49] Hou, L.; Pavan, W.J. Transcriptional and signaling regulation in neural crest stem cell-derived melanocyte development: do all roads lead to Mitf? *Cell Res.,* **2008**, *18*(12), 1163-1176.
[http://dx.doi.org/10.1038/cr.2008.303] [PMID: 19002157]

[50] Saldana-Caboverde, A.; Kos, L. Roles of endothelin signaling in melanocyte development and melanoma. *Pigment Cell Melanoma Res.,* **2010**, *23*(2), 160-170.
[http://dx.doi.org/10.1111/j.1755-148X.2010.00678.x] [PMID: 20128875]

[51] Sturm, R.A. A golden age of human pigmentation genetics. *Trends Genet.,* **2006**, *22*(9), 464-468.
[http://dx.doi.org/10.1016/j.tig.2006.06.010] [PMID: 16857289]

[52] Dupin, E.; Sommer, L. Neural crest progenitors and stem cells: from early development to adulthood. *Dev. Biol.,* **2012**, *366*(1), 83-95.
[http://dx.doi.org/10.1016/j.ydbio.2012.02.035] [PMID: 22425619]

[53] Duband, J.L. Diversity in the molecular and cellular strategies of epithelium-to-mesenchyme transitions: Insights from the neural crest. *Cell Adhes. Migr.,* **2010**, *4*(3), 458-482.
[http://dx.doi.org/10.4161/cam.4.3.12501] [PMID: 20559020]

[54] Gleason, B.C.; Crum, C.P.; Murphy, G.F. Expression patterns of MITF during human cutaneous embryogenesis: evidence for bulge epithelial expression and persistence of dermal melanoblasts. *J. Cutan. Pathol.,* **2008**, *35*(7), 615-622.
[http://dx.doi.org/10.1111/j.1600-0560.2007.00881.x] [PMID: 18312434]

[55] Zabierowski, S.E.; Fukunaga-Kalabis, M.; Li, L.; Herlyn, M. Dermis-derived stem cells: a source of epidermal melanocytes and melanoma? *Pigment Cell Melanoma Res.,* **2011**, *24*(3), 422-429.
[http://dx.doi.org/10.1111/j.1755-148X.2011.00847.x] [PMID: 21410654]

[56] Xiao, L.; Zhang, R.Z.; Zhu, W.Y. The distribution of melanocytes and the degradation of melanosomes in fetal hair follicles. *Micron,* **2019**, *119*, 109-116.
[http://dx.doi.org/10.1016/j.micron.2019.01.010] [PMID: 30711746]

[57] Opdecamp, K.; Nakayama, A.; Nguyen, M.T.; Hodgkinson, C.A.; Pavan, W.J.; Arnheiter, H. Melanocyte development *in vivo* and in neural crest cell cultures: crucial dependence on the Mitf basic-helix-loop-helix-zipper transcription factor. *Development,* **1997**, *124*(12), 2377-2386.
[PMID: 9199364]

[58] Widlund, H.R.; Fisher, D.E. Microphthalamia-associated transcription factor: a critical regulator of pigment cell development and survival. *Oncogene,* **2003**, *22*(20), 3035-3041.
[http://dx.doi.org/10.1038/sj.onc.1206443] [PMID: 12789278]

[59] Mollaaghababa, R.; Pavan, W.J. The importance of having your SOX on: role of SOX10 in the development of neural crest-derived melanocytes and glia. *Oncogene,* **2003**, *22*(20), 3024-3034.
[http://dx.doi.org/10.1038/sj.onc.1206442] [PMID: 12789277]

[60] Levy, C.; Khaled, M.; Fisher, D.E. MITF: master regulator of melanocyte development and melanoma oncogene. *Trends Mol. Med.,* **2006**, *12*(9), 406-414.
[http://dx.doi.org/10.1016/j.molmed.2006.07.008] [PMID: 16899407]

[61] Kawakami, A.; Fisher, D.E. The master role of microphthalmia-associated transcription factor in melanocyte and melanoma biology. *Lab. Invest.,* **2017**, *97*(6), 649-656.
[http://dx.doi.org/10.1038/labinvest.2017.9] [PMID: 28263292]

[62] Cronin, J.C.; Loftus, S.K.; Baxter, L.L.; Swatkoski, S.; Gucek, M.; Pavan, W.J. Identification and functional analysis of SOX10 phosphorylation sites in melanoma. *PLoS One,* **2018**, *13*(1), e0190834.
[http://dx.doi.org/10.1371/journal.pone.0190834] [PMID: 29315345]

<u>**CHAPTER 2**</u>

Melanophores and Smooth Muscles: A Comparative Perspective

Abstract: Melanophores or melanocytes, originated from the neural crest cells, contain melanosomes which are membrane-bound vesicles. Melanosomes are filled with dark coloured pigment called melanin, which has a crucial function in the biological color adaptation of vertebrates. Melanophore control *via* melanosome trafficking with microfilaments produce a variety of striking color pattern. Melanosome relaxation and contraction during pigment transfer is similar to the relaxation and contraction of smooth muscle cells. Studies have revealed that melanophores of all vertebrates including fish, amphibians, reptiles, mammals are functionally modified smooth muscle cells. The present chapter highlights the experimental based studies that have shown the comparison of melanophores with smooth muscle cells.

Keywords: Melanophores, Melanosomes, Microfilaments, Smooth muscles, Trafficking.

1. INTRODUCTION

Melanophores or melanocytes are the specified cells originated from neural crest cells, containing melanosomes, membrane-bound vesicles. Melanosomes are filled with dark colored pigment called melanin, which has a crucial function in the biological color adaptation of vertebrates. Melanophore control *via* melanosome trafficking with microfilaments produce a variety of striking color pattern. The physical and biochemical aspects of melanosome movement are the basis of mechanisms involved in physiological color change by melanophores. Melanosomes inside the melanophores aggregate or disperse if the host needs alteration in colour change, responding to environmental signals such as social interaction or camouflage [1, 2]. Fascinatingly, embryological, physiological and morphological evidence has disclosed that melanocytes or melanophores of all vertebrates including fishes, amphibians, birds and mammals are the modified smooth muscles [3, 4].

Furthermore, during melanophore contraction, melanin granules aggregate which is a visible similarity of an aggregation of colloidal particles which occurs during contraction of smooth muscles.The events specifically the biochemical events during the dispersion of melanosomes are similar to the relaxation of smooth muscles. Both the processes are the result of rising levels of cAMP and for their action, they require the presence of extracellular Ca^{2+} [3, 5]. A similar model of action involving the role of intracellular Ca^{2+} in CAMP elevation has been reported from our laboratory in the melanophore of teleost fish by Ali *et al.* [6] highlighting the similarity of melanophores with smooth muscle cells. In the present chapter, we have made a comparison between smooth muscles and melanophores with the support of various previously conducted studies.

2. MECHANISM OF SMOOTH MUSCLE CONTRACTION AND RELAXATION

To activate contraction in smooth muscle, ligands like hormones, and neurotransmitters bind to specific receptors. Consequently, the activation of a membrane phospholipid phosphatidylinositol 4, 5-biphosphate (PIP2) is the result of a rise in the activity of cellular phospholipase C *via* coupling to a G-protein. Diacylglycerol (DAG) and inositol 1, 4, 5-triphosphate (IP3) produced as second messengers by phospholipase C (PLC) from PIP2. IP3 binds to specific receptors and calcium (Ca^{2+}) releases. Later on, PKC is activated by DAG, which additionally phosphorylates specific target proteins. In smooth muscles, Ca^{2+} channels are phosphorylated by PKC that control cross-bridge cycling. A myosin light chain protein called MLC kinase is activated when Ca^{2+} attaches to calmodulin, a calcium modulated protein [7]. This step is the initiation of the muscle cell shortening along with actin *via* cross-bridge cycling. Ca^{2+} sensitizing mechanism maintained the condition of contraction, which is activated by ROCK, a Rho kinase protein. The activity of a motor protein, myosin is increased by ROCK *via* two mechanisms: First is the phosphorylation of MLC, which rises the activity of myosin II ATPase. As a result, many bundled and active myosins that are dynamic and active on many actin filaments, accelerate the filaments against each other leading to the shortening of actin fibres. The second mechanism involves the inactivation of MLC phosphatase, resulting in increased levels of phosphorylated MLC [7 - 9].

The relaxation process needs a reduced intracellular Ca^{2+} concentration and improved phosphatase activity of myosin light chain (MLC). Ca Mg- ATPases with Ca^{2+} / Na^+ exchangers present in plasma membrane, removes Ca^{2+} from the cytosol. Moreover, the entry of Ca^{2+} in the cell gets closed by the voltage-operated Ca^{2+} channels in the plasma membrane, leads to relaxation of smooth muscle cells [7]. It means that Ca^{2+} calmodulin-binding initiates the contractile activity of smooth muscles to activate myosin light chain phosphorylation. The mechanism of Ca^{2+} sensitization of contractile protein is signalled by Rho kinase pathway, in which inhibition of dephosphorylation of the light chain by myosin phosphatase occurred. Stimulation of myosin phosphatase and removal of Ca^{2+} from the cytoplasm initiates smooth muscle relaxation [7, 8].

3. MELANOPHORES AND SMOOTH MUSCLES: COMPARATIVE PERCEPTION

The first proof of the resemblance of melanophores with smooth muscle cells was presented by Spaeth in 1917 [3]. He has observed rhythmical pulsation in the isolated scale melanophores of *fundulus heteroclitus*. The observations followed by the core analysis of the melanophore responses and their behaviour to different impetus and their alikeness with smooth muscle cells represent melanophore as modified smooth muscle cells.

The biochemical events that occur during dispersion of melanophore are similar to the relaxation of smooth muscle, as a rise in the level of cAMP resulted in both these processes. Increased cAMP in smooth muscle causes relaxation. It is recognised that the rise in cAMP level starts the entry of Ca^{2+} from the cytosol to the inside of mitochondria and endoplasmic reticulum or out of smooth muscles. But, the dispersion of melanosome is progressed when Ca^{2+} is absent but extracellular Ca^{2+} is present [10]. The essential role of Ca^{2+} and MSH in melanophore's movement in two directions has been shown in Fig. (**1**). The inward movement of Ca^{2+} caused by the extracellular stimuli which may be either hormonal or mechanical activates phospholipase C (PLC). PLC promotes DAG (diacylglycerol) sensitive activation of PKC (protein kinase C) and inositol triphosphate (IP3) dependent release of Ca^{2+}. This further augments the influx of Ca^{2+} *via* voltage-dependent calcium channels, led to the aggregation of pigment.

Adenylyl cyclase stimulated by alpha MSH receptor raises the level of intracellular cAMP leading to dispersion of pigment by activating calcium pump which promotes Ca^{2+} out of the cell. The activity of melanocyte concentrating hormone (MSH) in melanocytes increases when intracellular Ca^{2+} is absent [11, 12], this is equivalent to the triggering by β- adrenergic receptors in smooth muscles. There is no clear mechanism known to show the actual route of melanosome translocation from the state of concentration to the state of dispersion. Nevertheless, the whole mechanism is extremely synchronized and needs several entities and factors.

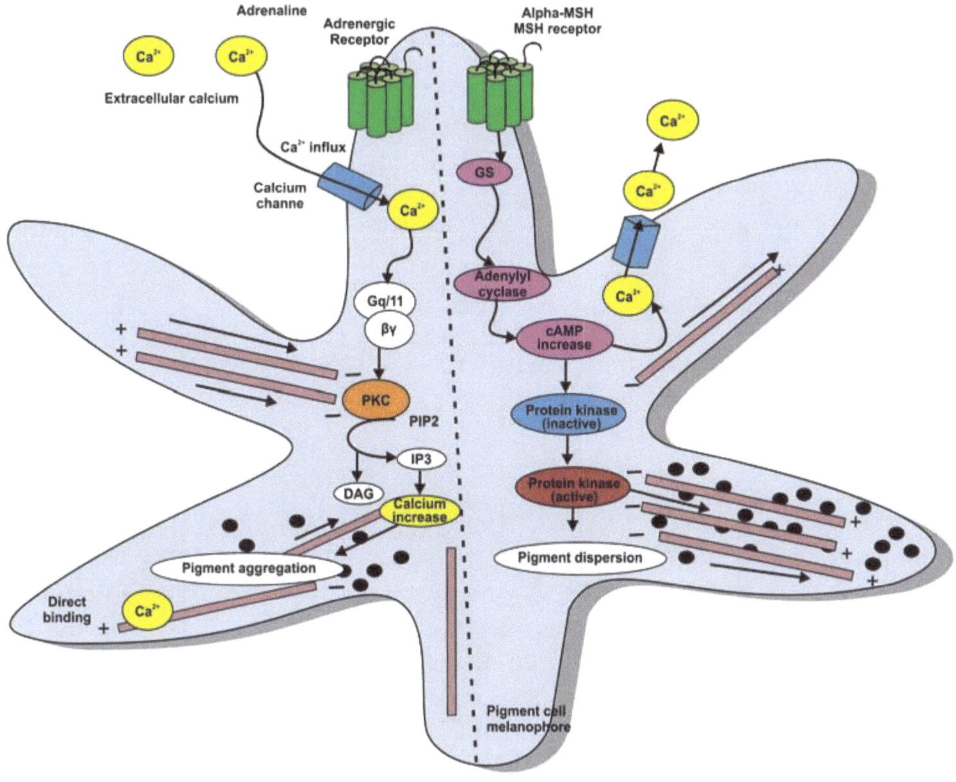

Fig. (1). Schematic representation of the role of Ca^{2+} and MSH in the bidirectional movement of melanophores.

4. EXPERIMENTS THAT REVEALS THE RESEMBLANCE OF MELANOPHORES WITH SMOOTH MUSCLE CELLS

Muscle cells are capable of responding to appropriate stimulation hence they are called 'excitable cells' However, the response to this contraction may differ. It can be either depolarization or electrical signals produced by the activity of neurons at the muscle cell's surface. But, a kind of muscle cells including smooth muscles respond to neuronal signals, they can also respond to direct mechanical and chemical stimulation [13]. In the same way, pigment cells have an innate capability of relocating pigment granules inside the cells in response to a given stimulus. Melanophore response to the stimuli is extremely synchronized in which there is receiving of external signals, thus causing a rigorous and proper response [14, 15]. This cell-to-cell communication largely governs the spread of signal molecules which may be either agonists or ligands, received *via* surface receptors present on recipient cells, leading to the usual movement of melanosomes in two directions, inside the melanophores or melanocytes [14, 15].

The highly prominent evidence of similarity between melanophores and smooth muscle in terms of physiology was provided by Franz in 1906 [16]. He demonstrated the resemblance between the response of the sphincter papillae in *Acanthias* and the frog's skin melanophores. Several workers have recorded the involvement of the nervous system and direct involvement of chromatophores, which have been widely accepted by many investigators and several reports published [17 - 20].

The resemblance of melanophores with smooth muscle cells can be explained based on the following heads:

4.1. Electrical Stimulation

Contraction of sphincter papillae of frog (*Rana*) and the eel was observed in response to the electrical stimulus. A similar contraction was reported in radial muscles of chromatophores of cephalopods [17]. Several species of teleosts have also shown such contractions. When the mounting medium has the proper strength, salt concentration, and duration of current, *Fundulus* melanophores invariably contract. In melanophores of *Hyla arborea* and *Rana esculenta*, similar results were recorded [21]. In line with the original observation of Brucke, Krukenberg [22] and Bert [23] have reported that excised pieces of chameleon skin produce lightning when their melanophores get contracted in response to direct faradic stimulation. In lower vertebrates including fishes, the nervous system has been developed to permit faster chromatic adaptation, hence the considerate division of the ANS (autonomic nervous system) is involved in melanophore's pigment aggregation.

4.2. Mechanical Stimulation

Powerful contractions have been reported in excised stomach and oesophagus pieces of fish and frog when it was gently stretched and pinched, provided the stimulus has not been so intense. Likewise, melanophores from Loligo skin pieces were expanded. Melanophores (aggregated) present in isolated fish scales of *Pterophyllum scalare*, an angelfish were mechanically compressed. By increasing mechanical force, melanophores disperse their pigment. The degree of melanin dispersion is directly proportional to the intensity of the external force [24].

4.3. Light Stimulation

It has been reported that the sphincter papillae of excised iris of some amphibians and fishes (teleost) responded to light. Similar light stimulation was observed in chromatophores of cephalopods, which was a direct outcome of relaxation and contraction of smooth muscle cells arranged radially [25]. Kargacin and Detwiler [26] have also reported light-evoked contraction in smooth muscles of the *Rana pipiens*, a frog. Generally, the movements of melanosomes in fishes are controlled by adrenergic nerves. Aggregation of melanosomes occurs in the presence of epinephrine and α-adrenergic blocking drugs inhibit the aggregation [27, 28]. In the presence of epinephrine, the cultured melanophores, which was light-sensitive also gets aggregated Dibenamine, an α-adrenergic blocking drug was found to inhibit the epinephrine responses but has not able to inhibit the light stimulated aggregation of melanosomes. These findings suggested that the light stimulus works directly on the phosphodiesterase enzyme as it controls the dynamics of melanosomes without adrenergic receptor mediation [28].

4.4. Chemical Stimulation

Various scientists have extensively studied the effects of different chemicals on pigment cells and muscle cells. Different neurotransmitters and other biogenic compounds have been analysed and it has been noticed that several receptors present on an effector cell for different neurotransmitters and hormones [15]. The various signals are read by the receptors on cells with raise or decline in levels of the intracellular second messenger. There are three-second messengers including which are known to take part in melanophore dynamics, Ca^{2+} (calcium), IP3 (1,4,5 tri-phosphate), cAMP (cyclic adenosine monophosphate). Fascinatingly, their role in smooth muscle contraction has also been described in various studies [29, 30].

As calcium is one of the very essential cation in terms of a variety of functions and has an important role in smooth muscle contraction and translocation of pigment. Several studies have supported the role of Ca^{2+} in smooth muscle contraction and pigment dynamics and translocation [31 - 42].

CONCLUSION

A complex and integrated array of events including the interaction of cytoskeletons, motor proteins, and its associated regulatory proteins are engaged in the regulation of normal responsiveness of pigment cells. The present chapter emphasized the function of melanophores and their dynamics that can well explain the dynamics of other cells such as muscle cells and *vice versa*. As cells communicate with another cell *via* their surface, thus cellular phenotypes are a versatile process that replicates the effect or influence of other cells. The study of these cellular systems would considerably contribute towards the understanding of both pathological and physiological events related to muscle and pigment cells.

REFERENCES

[1]   Ali, S.A.; Naaz, I. Comparative light and electron microscopic studies of dorsal skin melanophores of Indian toad, *Bufo melanostictus. J. Microsc. Ultrastruct,* **2014**, *2*(4), 230-235.
[http://dx.doi.org/10.1016/j.jmau.2014.07.002]

[2]   Ali, S.A.; Naaz, I. Understanding the ultrastructural aspects of berberine-induced skin-darkening activity in the toad, *Bufo melanostictus,* melanophores. *J Microsc Ultrastruct,* **2015**, *3*(4), 210-219.
[http://dx.doi.org/10.1016/j.jmau.2015.07.001] [PMID: 30023201]

[3]   Spaeth, R.A. Evidence proving melanophores as a disguised type of Smooth muscle cells. *J. Exp. Zool.,* **1917**, *20*(2), 193-215.
[http://dx.doi.org/10.1002/jez.1400200206]

[4]   Salim, S.; Ali, S.A. Melanophores: smooth muscle cells in disguise. In: *Current Basic and Pathological Approaches to the Function of Muscle Cells and Tissues - From Molecules to Humans*; InTech publishers, **2012**.
[http://dx.doi.org/10.5772/48256]

[5]   Eom, D.S.; Bain, E.J.; Patterson, L.B.; Grout, M.E.; Parichy, D.M. Long-distance communication by specialized cellular projections during pigment pattern development and evolution. *eLife,* **2015**, *4*, e12401.
[http://dx.doi.org/10.7554/eLife.12401] [PMID: 26701906]

[6]   Ali, S.A.; Ali, A.S.; Ovais, M.; Belsare, D.K. *In-vitro* effect of cyclic AMP on teleost melanophores. *Acad. Science Letters,* **1985**, *1985*(193), 294-297.

[7]   Webb, R.C. Smooth muscle contraction and relaxation. *Adv. Physiol. Educ.,* **2003**, *27*(1-4), 201-206.
[http://dx.doi.org/10.1152/advances.2003.27.4.201] [PMID: 14627618]

[8]   Castrucci, A.M.; Hadley, M.E.; Lebl, M.; Zechel, C.; Hruby, V.J. Melanocyte stimulating hormone and melanin concentration hormone may be structurally and evolutionarily related. *Regul. Pept.,* **1989**, *24*(1), 27-35.
[http://dx.doi.org/10.1016/0167-0115(89)90208-5] [PMID: 2544929]

[9]   Riento, K.; Ridley, A.J. Rocks: multifunctional kinases in cell behaviour. *Nat. Rev. Mol. Cell Biol.,* **2003**, *4*(6), 446-456.
[http://dx.doi.org/10.1038/nrm1128] [PMID: 12778124]

[10]   Vesely, D.L.; Hadley, M.E. Ionic requirements for melanophore stimulating hormone (MSH) action on melanophores. *Comp. Biochem. Physiol.,* **1979**, *62A*, 501-507.
[http://dx.doi.org/10.1016/0300-9629(79)90093-8]

[11]   Smith, D.C. Melanophore pulsations in the isolated scales of *fundulus heteroclitus. Proc. Natl. Acad. Sci. USA,* **1930**, *16*(6), 381-385.
[http://dx.doi.org/10.1073/pnas.16.6.381] [PMID: 16587586]

[12]   Hadley, M.E. *Endocrinology,* 5th ed; Printice Hall, **1988**.

[13]   Zhang, F.; Wang, L.P.; Boyden, E.S.; Deisseroth, K. Channelrhodopsin-2 and optical control of excitable cells. *Nat. Methods,* **2006**, *3*(10), 785-792.
[http://dx.doi.org/10.1038/nmeth936] [PMID: 16990810]

[14]   Aspengren, S.; Hedberg, D.; Wallin, M. Melanophores: a model system for neuronal transport and exocytosis? *J. Neurosci. Res.,* **2007**, *85*(12), 2591-2600.
[http://dx.doi.org/10.1002/jnr.21132] [PMID: 17149749]

[15]　Salim, S.; Ali, S.A. Vertebrate melanophores as potential model for drug discovery and development: a review. *Cell. Mol. Biol. Lett.,* **2011**, *16*(1), 162-200.
[http://dx.doi.org/10.2478/s11658-010-0044-y] [PMID: 21225472]

[16]　Franz, V. Beobachtungen am lebenden selachierauge. *Jenaische Zeitschr. f. Naturwiss., 41 (Nf.Bd. 34),* **1906**, 429-471.

[17]　Brucke, E. Untersuchungen uber den Farbenwechsel des afrikanischen chamaleons. *Denschr. Akad. Wiss. Wien, Mathnat. Kl,* **1852**, *4*, 179.

[18]　Pouchet, G. Color changes in crustaceans and fishes. *J. Anat. Physiol,* **1876**, *12*, 1-90.

[19]　Parker, G.H. *Animal Colour Changes and their Neurohumors*; Cambridge Univ. Press: Cambridge, U.K, **1948**.

[20]　Fujii, R. Cytophysiology of fish chromatophores. *Int. Rev. Cytol.,* **1993**, *143*, 191-255.
[http://dx.doi.org/10.1016/S0074-7696(08)61876-8]

[21]　Arch, W. *F. Derm. U. Syphilis.,* **1910**, *101*, 255.
[http://dx.doi.org/10.1007/BF01832761]

[22]　Krukenberg, C.F.W. Ueber die Mechanik des Farben wechseis bei Chamaeleon vulgaris, Cuv. *Vergleichend-physiologische Studien, Reihe 1, Abt. 3,* **1880**, 23-65.

[23]　Bert, P. Sur le mecanisme et les causes des changements de couleur chez le cam6l6on. *C. R,. Acad. Sei., Paris, torn.,* **1975**, *81*, 938-941.

[24]　Schliwa, M. Bereiter-Hahn. Pigment movements in fish melanophores: Morphological and physiological studies. *Cell Tissue Res.,* **1975**, *158*(1), 61-73.
[http://dx.doi.org/10.1007/BF00219951] [PMID: 1149080]

[25]　Hart, N.S.; Lisney, T.J.; Collin, S.P. Visual communication in Elasmobranchs. In: *Communication in Fishes*; Science publishers Inc: Enfield (NH), USA, **2004**; pp. 338-392.

[26]　Kargacin, G.J.; Detwiler, P.B. Light-evoked contraction of the photosensitive iris of the frog. *J. Neurosci.,* **1985**, *5*(11), 3081-3087.
[http://dx.doi.org/10.1523/JNEUROSCI.05-11-03081.1985] [PMID: 3932607]

[27]　Bagnara, J.T.; Hadley, M.E. *Chromatophores and color change: The comparative physiology of animal pigmentation*; Prentice-Hall, Inc: Englewood Cliffs, N. J., **1973**.

[28]　Wakamatu, Y. Light-sensitive fish melanophores in culture. *J. Exp. Zool.,* **1978**, *204*, 299-304.
[http://dx.doi.org/10.1002/jez.1402040218]

[29]　Kapoor, B.G.; Khanna, B. *Integument, dermal skeleton, coloration and pigment cells*; Ichthyology Handbook, Springer: Verlag Berlin Heidelberg, **2004**, pp. 65-73.

[30]　Thaler, C.D.; Haimo, L.T. Control of organelle transport in melanophores: regulation of Ca^{2+} and cAMP levels. *Cell Motil. Cytoskeleton,* **1992**, *22*(3), 175-184.
[http://dx.doi.org/10.1002/cm.970220305] [PMID: 1330333]

[31]　Karaki, H.; Ozaki, H.; Hori, M.; Mitsui-Saito, M.; Amano, K.; Harada, K.; Miyamoto, S.; Nakazawa, H.; Won, K.J.; Sato, K. Calcium movements, distribution, and functions in smooth muscle. *Pharmacol. Rev.,* **1997**, *49*(2), 157-230.
[PMID: 9228665]

[32]　Novales, R.R. The effect of the divalent cation ionophore A23187 on amphibian melanophores and iridophores. *J. Invest. Dermatol.,* **1977**, *69*(5), 446-450.
[http://dx.doi.org/10.1111/1523-1747.ep12511041] [PMID: 333033]

[33]　Tuma, M.C.; Gelfand, V.I. Molecular mechanisms of pigment transport in melanophores. *Pigment Cell Res.,* **1999**, *12*(5), 283-294.
[http://dx.doi.org/10.1111/j.1600-0749.1999.tb00762.x] [PMID: 10541038]

[34]   Fujii, R.; Fujii, Y. Mechanism of nervous control of fish melanophores. il role of divalent ions in the transmission at the melanin-aggregating nerve endings. *Zool. Mag,* **1965**, 74-351.

[35]   McNiven, M.A.; Porter, K.R. Chromatophores--models for studying cytomatrix translocations. *J. Cell Biol.,* **1984**, *99*(1 Pt 2), 152s-158s.
[http://dx.doi.org/10.1083/jcb.99.1.152s] [PMID: 6746727]

[36]   Schliwa, M. Permeabilized cell models for the study of granule transport in pigment cells. *Pigment Cell Res.,* **1987**, *1*(2), 65-68.
[http://dx.doi.org/10.1111/j.1600-0749.1987.tb00391.x] [PMID: 3333836]

[37]   Haimo, L.T.; Rozdzial, M.M. Lysed chromatophores: a model system for the study of bidirectional organelle transport. *Methods Cell Biol.,* **1989**, *31*, 3-24.
[http://dx.doi.org/10.1016/S0091-679X(08)61599-X] [PMID: 2779450]

[38]   Schliwa, M.; Bereiter-Hahn, J. Pigment movement in fish melanophores. III. The effects of colchicine and vinblastine. *Z. Zellforsch,* **1973**, *147*, 127-148.
[http://dx.doi.org/10.1007/BF00306604] [PMID: 4363098]

[39]   Murphy, D.B.; Tilney, L.G. The role of microtubules in the movement of pigment granules in teleost melanophores. *J. Cell Biol.,* **1974**, *61*(3), 757-779.
[http://dx.doi.org/10.1083/jcb.61.3.757] [PMID: 4836391]

[40]   Obika, M.; Negishi, S. Effects of hexylene glycol and nocodazole on microtubules and melanosome translocation in melanophores of the medaka, oryzias latipes. *J. Exp. Zool.,* **1985**, *235*, 55-63.
[http://dx.doi.org/10.1002/jez.1402350108]

[41]   Luby-Phelps, K.; Porter, K.R. The control of pigment migration in isolated erythrophores of *Holocentrus ascensionis* (Osbeck). II. The role of calcium. *Cell,* **1982**, *29*(2), 441-450.
[http://dx.doi.org/10.1016/0092-8674(82)90160-X] [PMID: 6811138]

[42]   Oshima, N.; Suzuki, M.; Yamaji, N.; Fujii, R. Pigment aggregation is triggered by an increase in free calcium ions within fish chromatophores. *Comp. Biochem. Physiol.,* **1988**, *91A*, 27-32.

CHAPTER 3

Melanogenesis: Mechanism and Factors Involved in Melanin Synthesis

Abstract: Vertebrate skin pigmentation is the phenotypic trait which is determined by a pigment, melanin; a biopolymer produced within epidermal melanocytes, packaged in specialized organelles called melanosomes by a process called melanogenesis. Eumelanin and pheomelanin are the two types of melanin formed within the melanocytes. The process of melanin production and its transfer to keratinocytes defines visible skin pigmentation. Various intrinsic factors including several genes involved in many signalling pathways such as SCF/KIT, neuregulin, endothelin, WNT, glutamatergic, adrenergic signalling pathways are involved in the process of melanogenesis. Along with the internal factors, some external factors including ultraviolet radiations, environmental pollutants and hormonal impregnation are also responsible for the increase of melanin synthesis. In the present chapter, we have discussed the biochemistry of the process of melanogenesis with a focus on a mechanism of melanin synthesis and the internal and external factors affecting melanogenesis.

Keywords: Melanin, Melanogenesis, Pigmentation, Signalling pathway, Ultraviolet radiation.

1. INTRODUCTION

Skin color is an important phenotypic trait of all vertebrates. In higher vertebrates, it is determined particularly by melanin which is a biopolymer synthesized within epidermal melanocytes, packaged in specialized organelles called melanosomes and this process of melanin synthesis is known as melanogenesis. Besides defining an essential phenotypic trait, melanin has an important role in photoprotection due to its capability of absorbing ultraviolet radiation [1]. Two types of melanin are synthesized within melanosomes: pheomelanin and eumelanin. Pheomelanin is light, red-yellow, and sulphur containing soluble pigment while eumelanin is dark, brown-black and insoluble. The types of melanin produced depend on the function of melanogenic enzymes and substrate availability. Both types of melanin are produced by the oxidation and polymerization of the common precursor L-tyrosine with the involvement of key enzyme of melanogenesis called tyrosinase [2 - 4].

Melanin produced by melanocytes is transferred to the surrounding cells of the epidermis called keratinocytes. Keratinocytes are the most abundant cells of the epidermis, they form around 95% of the total epidermal cell count. They are in close contact with melanocytes to take melanin by exo and endocytosis, in the form of enclosed melanin packages, melanosomes with the help of dendritic processes of melanocytes. This contact of melanocytes with keratinocytes is known as an epidermal melanin unit and it is crucial in that the skin will not appear pigmented until melanin is transferred to keratinocytes [5]. However, melanocytes contain melanin; they are located very deep within the epidermis to significantly affect the color of the skin. The difference in skin color is also attributed to the difference in the distribution and size of melanosomes. The size and quantity of the melanosomes are greater in the darker skin as compared to the lighter skin [6].

Constitutive skin pigmentation can be regulated by several intrinsic and extrinsic regulatory factors. Skin pigmentation involves three key cellular players; melanocytes and keratinocytes in the epidermis and fibroblasts in the dermis. These cells are very interactive and communicate with each other through various secreted factors including α-MSH, SCF, KGF and their receptors to regulate pigmentation. The signalling pathways involved during the process of melanogenesis coincide with microphthalmia-associated transcription factor (MITF), which are under the control of several genes of melanogenesis. Various environmental stimuli, such as UV radiation and environmental pollution can also affect skin pigmentation [5, 7]. So, in the present chapter, we have highlighted the main signalling pathways and the other key factors involved in melanogenesis and its regulation.

2. BIOCHEMISTRY OF MELANOGENESIS

Melanogenesis is a biochemical pathway responsible for melanin synthesis. It takes place in separate cytoplasmic organelles, melanosomes of melanocytes. Two types of melanin are produced: eumelanin and pheomelanin, their production mainly depends on substrate availability and function of melanogenesis enzymes. Visible skin pigmentation is preserved and depends on eumelanin content. It depends on the ratio of eumelanin to total melanin. Pheomelanin on the other hand, does not correlate with pigmentation; a similar amount of it is observed in dark and light skin. But the ratio of eumelanin to pheomelanin decides the color of the hair. Eumelanin is also considered to be more photoprotective than pheomelanin. Therefore, the risk of cancer in lighter skin is more prominent than the darker skin [8 - 10].

Melanin is produced from the precursor L-tyrosine, which gets hydroxylized to L-3-4-dihydroxyphenylalanine (DOPA) which is rapidly oxidized to DOPAquinone. When cysteine is present, DOPAquinone reacts with it, yielding 3- or 5-cysteinyl DOPAs, which is then oxidized and polymerized, producing yellow-red soluble pigment-pheomelanin. In the absence of cysteine, brown-black eumelanin is produced. DOPAquinone undergoes cyclization to DOPAchrome. The DOPAchrome loses carboxylic acid and generates 5, 6-dihydroxyindole (DHI), which is then oxidized and polymerized to form dark brown-black, DHI melanin. On the other hand, if DOPAchrome tautomerase (TRP2) is present, DOPachrome forms DHI-2-carboxylic acid (DHICA). Finally, tyrosinase-related protein 1 (TRP1) catalyzes further reactions obtaining a lighter brown color DHICA melanin. During melanogenesis, cytotoxic molecules, such as quinones and hydrogen peroxide are also produced as intermediate products [11 - 14] (Fig. **1**).

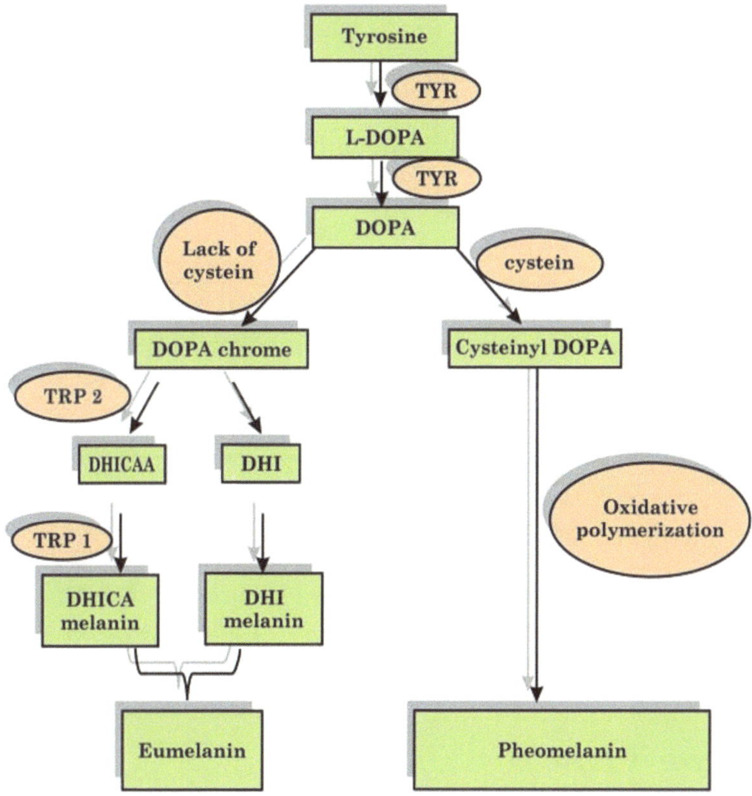

Fig (1). Biochemistry of melanin synthesis.

3. REGULATION OF MELANOGENESIS BY INTRINSIC FACTORS

Paracrine signals regulating the process of melanogenesis are delivered by the neighboring cells of melanocytes *i.e.* epidermal keratinocytes and dermal fibroblasts. Major signaling pathways involved are G-protein coupled receptors (GPCR) pathways (melanocortin receptors, endothelin receptors), tyrosine kinase receptors pathway (SCF/KIT signaling pathway, basic fibroblast growth factor (FGF) receptor and hepatocyte growth factors (HGF). The main pathway of melanogenesis is SCF/KIT pathway. Other pathways including adrenergic, neuregulin and glutamatergic pathways are considered as minor pathways.

3.1. G-Protein Coupled Receptors Pathways

3.1.1. CRF Pathway

A hypothalamic hormone called corticotrophin-releasing factor (CRF) controls the synthesis of pro-opiomelanocortin (POMC) in the pituitary. The synthesis of POMC is mediated by the binding of CRF to its type 1 receptors (CRF1) in the anterior pituitary. POMC will subsequently process to adrenocorticotropin (ACTH) and β lipotropin (βLPH). While melanocyte stimulating hormone (αMSH) is released due to the cleavage of ACTH and β- endorphin (βEND) produced from βLPH [15].

POMC, CRF, CRF1R and CRF2R are all expressed in human skin. Melanocytes, keratinocytes, and fibroblasts can produce and release CRF peptides. Isoforms of CRF1R can be expressed in the epidermis, whereas CRF2R can be expressed in hair follicles [16 - 18]. CRF proficiently induces the synthesis of POMC in epidermal melanocytes epidermal keratinocytes and dermal fibroblasts *via* signaling involving phospholipase C, adenylate cyclise and calcium channels, resulting in the activation of certain transcription factors including cAMP response element-binding protein (CREB), activator protein (AP-1), and nuclear factor kappa-light-chain-enhancer of activated B cells (NF-κB). The resultant peptides after processing of POMC maintain the modulatory activity of CRF on human skin pigmentation in an autocrine or paracrine way [19 - 22].

3.1.2. POMC Derived Peptides

The two melanocortin peptides involved in melanogenesis in human beings are melanocyte-stimulating hormone (αMSH) and adrenocorticotropin hormone (ACTH) [23]. Both αMSH and ACTH are derived from the same precursor, POMC by proteolytic cleavage. POMC and other melanocortin peptides were originally discovered in the anterior pituitary but are also expressed and secreted by epidermal melanocytes, keratinocytes, and Langerhan's cells [1, 24, 25]. αMSH is a 13 amino acid peptide regulating skin pigmentation *via* binding to melanocortin 1 receptor (MC1R). The binding of αMSH to MC1R brings the G protein-dependent activation of adenylate cyclise elevating intracellular cAMP and the subsequent stimulation of protein kinase A (PKA). While increasing cAMP, CREB activates by phosphorylation and eventually stimulates the transcription of MITF gene [26, 27]. ACTH is a 39 amino acid peptide having a cleavable sequence of αMSH in amino-terminal position and it is also a ligand of MC1R. Similar to αMSH, βMSH also activates adenylate cyclase which results in increasing the intracellular cAMP level, leading to regulate the MITF transcription [27, 28].

In addition to POMC derived ACTH, αMSH, βMSH, β-endorphin is also a modulator at the hair follicles. β- endorphin is a 31 amino acid peptide shown to regulate melanogenesis through G protein coupled opiate μ-receptor present at the surface of skin melanocytes. It regulates melanogenesis, melanocyte proliferation and dendricity *via* PKC (protein kinase C) mediated mechanism as well as modulate the melanocyte biology at the hair follicle [29, 30].

3.1.3. Endothelin Signaling Pathway

Endothelin-1 (EDN1) binds to the endothelin receptor type B (ETB), a G-protein coupled receptor, activates phospholipase Cγ (PLCγ), increases the hydrolysis of phosphatidylinositol 4, 5 biphosphate (PIP2) and finally generating Diacylglycerol (DAG) and inositol triphosphate (IP3). DAG stimulates the activation of PKC and IP3 increases the intracellular concentration of Ca^{2+}. Production of EDN1 in human skin and the expression level of tyrosinase is enhanced by UVB radiation leading to UVB induced pigmentation [31 - 33].

3.1.4. WNT Signaling Pathway

Wingless type MMTV integration site (WNT) represents a member of the family of cysteine rich lipoglycoproteins, having function in ontogeny and homeostasis. It binds to class frizzled receptors (FZD) and activating the intracellular cascade of events with (canonical form) or without (non-canonical form) the involvement of β-catenin, a transcription regulator [34]. WNT binds to FZD, which leads to the inhibition of glycogen synthase kinase 3β (GSK3β). β-catenin is then transferred to the nucleus and regulates MITF transcription. Additionally, both WNT1 and WNT3A have their roles in the development and differentiation of pigment cells from neural crest cells and also act on melanoblasts to maintain expression of

MITF [35 - 38]. Dickkopf 1 (DKK1) secreted by human palmo-plantar fibroblasts is an inhibitor of WNT pathway. It inhibits melanocyte function through the downregulation of β-catenin, MITF, PKC3 and GSK3β expression [39].

3.1.5. Glutamatergic and Adrenergic Signaling Pathways

Glutamatergic signaling involving glutamate receptors including glutamate receptor 2 (GluR2, AMPA receptor), glutamate receptor 4 (GluR4, AMPA receptor), NMDA receptors 2A and 2C (NMDAR2A and NMDAR2C) promote transcriptional regulation of MITF [40].

Epinephrine and norepinephrine produced by keratinocytes bind to the adrenergic receptors present on neighboring melanocytes [41]. Epinephrine and norepinephrine are catecholamines synthesized from a precursor of melanin, L-dihyroxyphenylalanine (L-DOPA) [12]. α 1-adrenergic receptors expressed in human melanocytes coupled with phospholipase C (PLC) produce IP3 and DAG from phosphatidylinositol 4,5-bisphosphate (PIP2). Then, IP3 increases the intracellular Ca2+ concentration and DAG activates PKCβ, which in turn releases tyrosine and other related proteins [42, 43].

4. TYROSINE KINASE RECEPTORS PATHWAY

4.1. SCF/KIT Pathway

Stem cell factor (SCF or KIT ligand) is a keratinocyte derived growth factor secreted by keratinocytes and fibroblasts [3]. It is the specific ligand of the tyrosine-protein kinase receptor. It binds to the KIT domain to provoke the receptor dimerization leading to its activation. Receptor in turn phosphorylates and binds to GRB2 (growth factor receptor-bound protein 2), SHC (Src homology domain), and guanine nucleotide exchange factor SOS (son of sevenless) resulting in phosphorylation of RAS (a small GTP binding protein). RAS in turn activates MAPK pathway. This chain of activation persuades phosphorylation of MITF, which allows the consequent transcription of melanogenic enzymes including TYR, TYRP1 and TYRP2. In addition to the melanogenic genes, several other genes are downregulated by MITF [44 - 46].

4.2. bFGF and HGF Signalling Pathway

Basic fibroblast growth factor also called as FGF-2 acts on melanocyte proliferation and melanin synthesis but is secreted by keratinocytes [47]. When bFGF binds to its receptor FGFR present on melanocyte, it leads to the activation of MAPK pathway [48, 49]. Similarly, hepatocyte growth factors (HGF) are secreted by keratinocytes, which bind to its receptor c-Met on melanocytes and can lead to the activation of MAPK pathway [50 - 52].

4.3. Neuregulin Pathway and BMP Pathway

NRG1 (neuregulin 1) is a factor secreted by fibroblasts and binds to the class I receptor tyrosine kinase particularly ERBB3 and ERBB4 (erb-b2 receptor kinase 3 and 4) and ultimately leads to the activation of phosphatidylinositol-3-kinase and MAPK pathway [53].

Bone morphogenetic proteins (BMPs), a class of signaling molecules have an important role in the regulation of skin hyperpigmentation, epidermal homeostasis. BMP6 is specifically involved in the stimulation of melanogenesis through upregulating tyrosinase expression and its activity. On the other hand, BMP4 affects melanogenesis *via* downregulating the expression of TYR, TYRP1, TYRP2, MC1R, PKC-β [54, 55].

5. PACKAGING OF MELANIN AND MELANOSOMES TRANSFER

5.1. Formation of Melanosomes

Melanin is produced inside an intracellular elliptical organelle called melanosome with the melanocytes. Melanosomes are the tissue-specific lysosome related organelles specific for the synthesis and storage of melanin. The origin of melanosomes is controversial; studies have suggested its origin from endoplasmic reticulum or endosomes [56, 57]. Melanosome maturation occurs in four stages. In stage I, their structure is similar to vascular domain of early endosomes in which intraluminal vesicles (ILVs) are present with the deposition of fibrils of pigment cell specific protein (PMEL17). PMEL17 is responsible for the elliptical shape of melanosomes. In stage II, the ellipsoidal form of melanosomes are morphologically changed due to the PMEL17 fibrils organized after cleavage of PMEL17 and release of Mα moiety which is formed from Mβ membrane fragment. Stage I and stage II melanosomes are called as premelanosomes in which melanin is not deposited; it is deposited in PMEL17 fibrils of stage III melanosomes. Fully filled melanosomes with melanin are the characteristic of stage IV. From stage II to IV, melanogenesis proteins including TYR, TYRP1 and TYRP2 are addressed to melanosomes [58 - 61].

In addition to PMEL17, several other proteins like OA1, MART1, SLC45A2, are involved in melanosome biogenesis. OA1 (ocular albinism 1) is the G-protein coupled receptor for L-DOPA and tyrosine. Mutation in OA1 causes ocular albinism. Albinism is the condition in which there is an alteration in pigment synthesis as a result of gene mutation through various mechanisms. There are two categories of albinism; one is oculocutaneous albinism (OCA) in which pigment synthesis is dysfunctional in skin, hair, and eye. Other category of albinism is ocular albinism in which only the eye is affected [62 - 64].

5.2. Melanogenic Enzyme Delivery into Melanosomes

In order to synthesize melanin, melanogenic enzymes have to be delivered into melanosomes. Two pathways are involved in protein transport from the early endosome to melanosomes. One pathway is mediated by adaptor-related protein complex mainly AP-3 and AP-1 and the other pathway is mediated by biogenesis of lysosomal organelles complex 1 and 2 (BLOC-1 and BLOC-2). Many of the genes coding for AP and BLOC subunits are transcriptional controlled by MITF. AP-3 (Adaptor protein complex) is the heterotetrameric protein complex. AP-3 exists as ubiquitous and as tissue specific isoforms. The ubiquitous expressed AP-3 allows the transport of tyrosinase from endosomes to melanosomes. Additionally, AP-1 allows the organization of tyrosinase and tyrosinase-related protein-1 by employing the microtubule motor protein KIF13A [57, 65].

Other protein complexes involved in assembling of the melanogenic enzyme into melanosomes are BLOC proteins. BLOC 1 is a complex having multi-subunits including BLOS1, BLOS2, BLOS3, cappuccino, muted, paladin, snapin and dysbindin. BLOC1 allows the delivery of ATP7A, a copper carrier that is essential for tyrosinase activity, to the melanosomes. BLOC2 on the other hand, having three subunits leads to the impaired delivery of tyrosinase and tyrosinase-related protein-1.BLOC3 is another complex of this protein family but its role in melanogenesis is not clear [66, 67].

5.3. Melanosome Transfer to Keratinocytes

Packaged melanin is transferred from melanocytes to neighboring keratinocytes to ensure skin pigmentation. The exact mechanism of melanosome transfer to keratinocytes is not that clear. Indeed, various mechanisms are proposed including exocytosis, cytophagocytosis, fusion of plasma membrane, transfer by membrane vesicles, through cytoplasmic projections called filopodia [68, 69]. Myosin 10 (MYO10) plays an important role in the regulation of melanosome transfer , decreases the number of filopodia and melanosome transfer to keratinocytes as observed in cultured melanocytes [70].

Protease-activated receptor 2 (PAR2) is involved in the regulation of melanosomes from melanocytes to keratinocytes. PAR2 is a unique family of G-protein coupled seven-transmembrane receptors. It is activated by proteolytic cleavage of its extra cellular N-terminal moiety. PAR2 is expressed in epidermal keratinocytes [71, 72]. Sharlow *et al.* [73] have demonstrated that activation of PAR2 increases phagocytosis of melanosomes by keratinocytes *via* Rho-dependent mechanism. Keratinocyte growth factor (KGF) is another signaling protein involved in the stimulation of melanosome transfer. It is secreted by human fibroblasts as a paracrine factor. KGF binds to keratinocyte growth factor receptor (KGFR), causing intracellular events that result in the activation of actin polymerization and enhancing phagocytosis of melanosomes [74].

6. REGULATION OF MELANOGENESIS BY EXTERNAL ENVIRONMENT

As the skin is a type of organ of our body which is in continuous contact with the external environment and is exposed to different environmental aggressions that affects epidermal pigmentation. The major external factors that affect skin pigmentation are:

6.1. Solar Ultraviolet Radiation

UV radiation causes the induction of several pathways of melanogenesis which results in increased production of melanin. Irradiation of UV increases the secretion of αMSH in keratinocytes followed by induction of DNA damage which causes p53-mediated transcription of POMC precursor genes [75]. It also regulates the expression of MITF and MITF regulated proteins including TYR, TYRP1, TYRP2, MART-1, PMEL17 resulting in increased melanin production [76, 77]. It also induces PAR2 expression that helps in the transfer and distribution of melanosomes [78]. UV irradiation also regulates the expression of interleukin-1 and endothelin- 1 in keratinocytes. Interleukin-1 activates the autocrine secretion of αMSH, ACTH, bFGF [79]. Several other melanogenic factors including SGF and NGF are also induced by UV irradiation [80].

In addition to this transcriptional regulation, UV exposure also induces the increase in intracellular Ca^{++} in melanocytes *via* calcium selective ORAI1, which results in increased transfer of melanosomes to keratinocytes *via* a mechanism mediated by filopodia and myosin-10 [81]. UV irradiation causes melanocytes to release PGE2 prostaglandin leading to tyrosinase modulation through EP3 and EP4 subtypes of G-protein coupled receptors that regulate cAMP/PKA signaling pathway [82]. Some studies have described the activation of melanogenesis *via* UVA involved phototransduction involving a light-sensitive receptor protein called rhodopsin (OPN2) [83].

6.2. Environmental Pollution

Due to industrial activities including the manufacture of herbicides and pesticides, incineration and many toxic contaminants are released into the environment and cause various skin pigmentation problems such as hyperpigmentation [84]. Pollutants like polycyclic aromatic hydrocarbon (PAH) triggers the aryl hydrocarbon receptor (AHR) and also induce a signaling pathway [85, 86]. Some workers showed that activation of AHR pathway induces the activity of tyrosinase leading to an increase in melanin production [87]. Besides activation of melanogenesis, some pollutants are able to inhibit the process of melanogenesis. Nuclear factor E2-related factor 2 (NRF2) involved in oxidative stress response stimulated by exposure to UV radiation and toxic pollutants, inhibits melanogenesis [88].

6.3. Hormonal Fluctuations

There is a known impact of some hormones on skin pigmentation and this may occur during hormonal changes. Besides αMSH, pigmentation is also controlled by other cellular hormones such as estrogen and progesterone. However, there is no receptor for estrogen and progesterone on human melanocytes but they increase melanin synthesis *via* non classical membrane bound receptors. Estrogen stimulates melanogenesis through G-protein coupled estrogen receptor and progesterone increases melanin synthesis *via* progestin and adipoQ receptor 7 [89].

CONCLUSION

The present chapter highlights the modulatory events underlying the regulation of skin pigmentation. Deregulation of pigmentation causes skin disorders affecting the patient's quality of life with psychosocial impact. Specific mutations of genes involved in melanogenesis causes pathological modification of skin pigmentation leading to various syndromes. Thus, it is important to understand the interrelated processes involved in melanogenesis including intracellular pathways. Regulation of melanogenesis is also driven by the external environment like UV radiation, environmental pollutants, and the physiological status of the organisms like hormonal changes.

REFERENCES

[1]   Lin, J.Y.; Fisher, D.E. Melanocyte biology and skin pigmentation. *Nature,* **2007**, *445*(7130), 843-850.
[http://dx.doi.org/10.1038/nature05660] [PMID: 17314970]

[2]   Costin, G.E.; Hearing, V.J. Human skin pigmentation: melanocytes modulate skin color in response to stress. *FASEB J.,* **2007**, *21*(4), 976-994.
[http://dx.doi.org/10.1096/fj.06-6649rev] [PMID: 17242160]

[3]   Cichorek, M.; Wachulska, M.; Stasiewicz, A.; Tymińska, A. Skin melanocytes: biology and development. *Postepy Dermatol. Alergol.,* **2013**, *30*(1), 30-41.
[http://dx.doi.org/10.5114/pdia.2013.33376] [PMID: 24278043]

[4]   Maranduca, M.A.; Branisteanu, D.; Serban, D.N.; Branisteanu, D.C.; Stoleriu, G.; Manolache, N.; Serban, I.L. Synthesis and physiological implications of melanic pigments. *Oncol. Lett.,* **2019**, *17*(5), 4183-4187.
[http://dx.doi.org/10.3892/ol.2019.10071] [PMID: 30944614]

[5]   Virador, V.M.; Muller, J.; Wu, X.; Abdel-Malek, Z.A.; Yu, Z.X.; Ferrans, V.J.; Kobayashi, N.; Wakamatsu, K.; Ito, S.; Hammer, J.A.; Hearing, V.J. Influence of α-melanocyte-stimulating hormone and ultraviolet radiation on the transfer of melanosomes to keratinocytes. *FASEB J.,* **2002**, *16*(1), 105-107.
[http://dx.doi.org/10.1096/fj.01-0518fje] [PMID: 11729101]

[6]   Bonaventure, J.; Domingues, M.J.; Larue, L. Cellular and molecular mechanisms controlling the migration of melanocytes and melanoma cells. *Pigment Cell Melanoma Res.,* **2013**, *26*(3), 316-325.
[http://dx.doi.org/10.1111/pcmr.12080] [PMID: 23433358]

[7]   D'Mello, S.A.; Finlay, G.J.; Baguley, B.C.; Askarian-Amiri, M.E. Signaling Pathways in Melanogenesis. *Int. J. Mol. Sci.,* **2016**, *17*(7), E1144.
[http://dx.doi.org/10.3390/ijms17071144] [PMID: 27428965]

[8]   Seiji, M.; Fitzpatrick, T.B. The reciprocal relationship between melanization and tyrosinase activity in melanosomes (melanin granules). *J. Biochem.,* **1961**, *49*, 700-706.
[http://dx.doi.org/10.1093/oxfordjournals.jbchem.a127360] [PMID: 13749805]

[9]   Fitzpatrick, T.B.; Miyamoto, M.; Ishikawa, K. The evolution of concepts of melanin biology. *Arch. Dermatol.,* **1967**, *96*(3), 305-323.
[http://dx.doi.org/10.1001/archderm.1967.01610030083015] [PMID: 5341550]

[10]   Ito, S.; Wakamatsu, K. Diversity of human hair pigmentation as studied by chemical analysis of eumelanin and pheomelanin. *J. Eur. Acad. Dermatol. Venereol.,* **2011**, *25*(12), 1369-1380.
[http://dx.doi.org/10.1111/j.1468-3083.2011.04278.x] [PMID: 22077870]

[11]   del Marmol, V.; Beermann, F. Tyrosinase and related proteins in mammalian pigmentation. *FEBS Lett.,* **1996**, *381*(3), 165-168.
[http://dx.doi.org/10.1016/0014-5793(96)00109-3] [PMID: 8601447]

[12]   Slominski, A.; Tobin, D.J.; Shibahara, S.; Wortsman, J. Melanin pigmentation in mammalian skin and its hormonal regulation. *Physiol. Rev.,* **2004**, *84*(4), 1155-1228.
[http://dx.doi.org/10.1152/physrev.00044.2003] [PMID: 15383650]

[13]   Simon, J.D.; Peles, D.; Wakamatsu, K.; Ito, S. Current challenges in understanding melanogenesis: bridging chemistry, biological control, morphology, and function. *Pigment Cell Melanoma Res.,* **2009**, *22*(5), 563-579.
[http://dx.doi.org/10.1111/j.1755-148X.2009.00610.x] [PMID: 19627559]

[14]   Hearing, V.J. Determination of melanin synthetic pathway. *J. Invest. Dermatol.,* **2011**, *131*, 8-11.

[http://dx.doi.org/10.1038/skinbio.2011.4]

[15]   Slominski, A.; Zbytek, B.; Zmijewski, M.; Slominski, R.M.; Kauser, S.; Wortsman, J.; Tobin, D.J. Corticotropin releasing hormone and the skin. *Front. Biosci.,* **2006,** *11*(11), 2230-2248.
[http://dx.doi.org/10.2741/1966] [PMID: 16720310]

[16]   Ito, N.; Ito, T.; Kromminga, A.; Bettermann, A.; Takigawa, M.; Kees, F.; Straub, R.H.; Paus, R. Human hair follicles display a functional equivalent of the hypothalamic-pituitary-adrenal axis and synthesize cortisol. *FASEB J.,* **2005,** *19*(10), 1332-1334.
[http://dx.doi.org/10.1096/fj.04-1968fje] [PMID: 15946990]

[17]   Slominski, A.; Zbytek, B.; Pisarchik, A.; Slominski, R.M.; Zmijewski, M.A.; Wortsman, J. CRH functions as a growth factor/cytokine in the skin. *J. Cell. Physiol.,* **2006,** *206*(3), 780-791.
[http://dx.doi.org/10.1002/jcp.20530] [PMID: 16245303]

[18]   Slominski, A.; Wortsman, J.; Paus, R.; Elias, P.M.; Tobin, D.J.; Feingold, K.R. Skin as an endocrine organ: implications for its function. *Drug Discov. Today Dis. Mech.,* **2008,** *5*(2), 137-144.
[http://dx.doi.org/10.1016/j.ddmec.2008.04.004] [PMID: 19492070]

[19]   Slominski, A.; Zbytek, B.; Semak, I.; Sweatman, T.; Wortsman, J. CRH stimulates POMC activity and corticosterone production in dermal fibroblasts. *J. Neuroimmunol.,* **2005,** *162*, 97-102.
[http://dx.doi.org/10.1016/j.jneuroim.2005.01.014]

[20]   Slominski, A.; Zbytek, B.; Szczesniewski, A.; Semak, I.; Kaminski, J.; Sweatman, T.; Wortsman, J. CRH stimulation of corticosteroids production in melanocytes is mediated by ACTH. *Am. J. Physiol. Endocrinol. Metab.,* **2005,** *288*, E701-E706.
[http://dx.doi.org/10.1152/ajpendo.00519.2004]

[21]   Rousseau, K.; Kauser, S.; Pritchard, L.E.; Warhurst, A.; Oliver, R.L.; Slominski, A.; Wei, E.T.; Thody, A.J.; Tobin, D.J.; White, A. Proopiomelanocortin (POMC), the ACTH/melanocortin precursor, is secreted by human epidermal keratinocytes and melanocytes and stimulates melanogenesis. *FASEB J.,* **2007,** *21*(8), 1844-1856.
[http://dx.doi.org/10.1096/fj.06-7398com] [PMID: 17317724]

[22]   Zmijewski, M.A.; Slominski, A.T. Emerging role of alternative splicing of CRF1 receptor in CRF signaling. *Acta Biochim. Pol.,* **2010,** *57*(1), 1-13.
[http://dx.doi.org/10.18388/abp.2010_2366] [PMID: 20234885]

[23]   McLeod, S.D.; Smith, C.; Mason, R.S. Stimulation of tyrosinase in human melanocytes by pro-opiomelanocortin-derived peptides. *J. Endocrinol.,* **1995,** *146*(3), 439-447.
[http://dx.doi.org/10.1677/joe.0.1460439] [PMID: 7595139]

[24]   Morhenn, V.B. The physiology of scratching: involvement of proopiomelanocortin gene-coded proteins in Langerhans cells. *Prog. Neuro. Endo. Immunol.,* **1991,** *4*, 265-267.

[25]   Tsatmali, M.; Ancans, J.; Thody, A.J. Melanocyte function and its control by melanocortin peptides. *J. Histochem. Cytochem.,* **2002,** *50*(2), 125-133.
[http://dx.doi.org/10.1177/002215540205000201] [PMID: 11799132]

[26]   Lee, A.Y.; Noh, M. The regulation of epidermal melanogenesis *via* cAMP and/or PKC signaling pathways: insights for the development of hypopigmenting agents. *Arch. Pharm. Res.,* **2013,** *36*(7), 792-801.
[http://dx.doi.org/10.1007/s12272-013-0130-6] [PMID: 23604723]

[27]   Wolf Horrell, E.M.; Boulanger, M.C.; D'Orazio, J.A. Melanocortin 1 Receptor: Structure, Function, and Regulation. *Front. Genet.,* **2016,** *7*, 95.
[http://dx.doi.org/10.3389/fgene.2016.00095] [PMID: 27303435]

[28]   Wikberg, J.E.; Muceniece, R.; Mandrika, I.; Prusis, P.; Lindblom, J.; Post, C.; Skottner, A. New aspects on the melanocortins and their receptors. *Pharmacol. Res.,* **2000,** *42*(5), 393-420.
[http://dx.doi.org/10.1006/phrs.2000.0725] [PMID: 11023702]

[29]   Kauser, S.; Schallreuter, K.U.; Thody, A.J.; Gummer, C.; Tobin, D.J. Regulation of human epidermal

melanocyte biology by beta-endorphin. *J. Invest. Dermatol.,* **2003**, *120*(6), 1073-1080.
[http://dx.doi.org/10.1046/j.1523-1747.2003.12242.x] [PMID: 12787137]

[30]　Kauser, S.; Thody, A.J.; Schallreuter, K.U.; Gummer, C.L.; Tobin, D.J. beta-Endorphin as a regulator of human hair follicle melanocyte biology. *J. Invest. Dermatol.,* **2004**, *123*(1), 184-195.
[http://dx.doi.org/10.1111/j.0022-202X.2004.22724.x] [PMID: 15191559]

[31]　Yada, Y.; Higuchi, K.; Imokawa, G. Effects of endothelins on signal transduction and proliferation in human melanocytes. *J. Biol. Chem.,* **1991**, *266*(27), 18352-18357.
[PMID: 1917960]

[32]　Imokawa, G.; Kobayashi, T.; Miyagishi, M.; Higashi, K.; Yada, Y. The role of endothelin-1 in epidermal hyperpigmentation and signaling mechanisms of mitogenesis and melanogenesis. *Pigment Cell Res.,* **1997**, *10*(4), 218-228.
[http://dx.doi.org/10.1111/j.1600-0749.1997.tb00488.x] [PMID: 9263329]

[33]　Imokawa, G.; Ishida, K. Inhibitors of intracellular signaling pathways that lead to stimulated epidermal pigmentation: perspective of anti-pigmenting agents. *Int. J. Mol. Sci.,* **2014**, *15*(5), 8293-8315.
[http://dx.doi.org/10.3390/ijms15058293] [PMID: 24823877]

[34]　Schulte, G. International Union of Basic and Clinical Pharmacology. LXXX. The class Frizzled receptors. *Pharmacol. Rev.,* **2010**, *62*(4), 632-667.
[http://dx.doi.org/10.1124/pr.110.002931] [PMID: 21079039]

[35]　Takeda, K.; Yasumoto, K.; Takada, R.; Takada, S.; Watanabe, K.; Udono, T.; Saito, H.; Takahashi, K.; Shibahara, S. Induction of melanocyte-specific microphthalmia-associated transcription factor by Wnt-3a. *J. Biol. Chem.,* **2000**, *275*(19), 14013-14016.
[http://dx.doi.org/10.1074/jbc.C000113200] [PMID: 10747853]

[36]　Jin, E.J.; Erickson, C.A.; Takada, S.; Burrus, L.W. Wnt and BMP signaling govern lineage segregation of melanocytes in the avian embryo. *Dev. Biol.,* **2001**, *233*(1), 22-37.
[http://dx.doi.org/10.1006/dbio.2001.0222] [PMID: 11319855]

[37]　Steingrímsson, E.; Copeland, N.G.; Jenkins, N.A. Melanocytes and the microphthalmia transcription factor network. *Annu. Rev. Genet.,* **2004**, *38*, 365-411.
[http://dx.doi.org/10.1146/annurev.genet.38.072902.092717] [PMID: 15568981]

[38]　Dunn, K.J.; Brady, M.; Ochsenbauer-Jambor, C.; Snyder, S.; Incao, A.; Pavan, W.J. WNT1 and WNT3a promote expansion of melanocytes through distinct modes of action. *Pigment Cell Res.,* **2005**, *18*(3), 167-180.
[http://dx.doi.org/10.1111/j.1600-0749.2005.00226.x] [PMID: 15892713]

[39]　Yamaguchi, Y.; Passeron, T.; Watabe, H.; Yasumoto, K.; Rouzaud, F.; Hoashi, T.; Hearing, V.J. The effects of dickkopf 1 on gene expression and Wnt signaling by melanocytes: mechanisms underlying its suppression of melanocyte function and proliferation. *J. Invest. Dermatol.,* **2007**, *127*(5), 1217-1225.
[http://dx.doi.org/10.1038/sj.jid.5700629] [PMID: 17159916]

[40]　Hoogduijn, M.J.; Hitchcock, I.S.; Smit, N.P.; Gillbro, J.M.; Schallreuter, K.U.; Genever, P.G. Glutamate receptors on human melanocytes regulate the expression of MiTF. *Pigment Cell Res.,* **2006**, *19*(1), 58-67.
[http://dx.doi.org/10.1111/j.1600-0749.2005.00284.x] [PMID: 16420247]

[41]　Schallreuter, K.U.; Wood, J.M.; Lemke, R.; LePoole, C.; Das, P.; Westerhof, W.; Pittelkow, M.R.; Thody, A.J. Production of catecholamines in the human epidermis. *Biochem. Biophys. Res. Commun.,* **1992**, *189*(1), 72-78.
[http://dx.doi.org/10.1016/0006-291X(92)91527-W] [PMID: 1360208]

[42]　Schallreuter, K.U.; Körner, C.; Pittelkow, M.R.; Swanson, N.N.; Gardner, M.L. The induction of the alpha-1-adrenoceptor signal transduction system on human melanocytes. *Exp. Dermatol.,* **1996**, *5*(1), 20-23.
[http://dx.doi.org/10.1111/j.1600-0625.1996.tb00088.x] [PMID: 8624607]

[43]   Bae-Harboe, Y.S.; Park, H.Y. Tyrosinase: a central regulatory protein for cutaneous pigmentation. *J. Invest. Dermatol.,* **2012,** *132*(12), 2678-2680.
[http://dx.doi.org/10.1038/jid.2012.324] [PMID: 23187110]

[44]   Hemesath, T.J.; Price, E.R.; Takemoto, C.; Badalian, T.; Fisher, D.E. MAP kinase links the transcription factor Microphthalmia to c-Kit signalling in melanocytes. *Nature,* **1998,** *391*(6664), 298-301.
[http://dx.doi.org/10.1038/34681] [PMID: 9440696]

[45]   Bertolotto, C.; Buscà, R.; Abbe, P.; Bille, K.; Aberdam, E.; Ortonne, J.P.; Ballotti, R. Different cis-acting elements are involved in the regulation of TRP1 and TRP2 promoter activities by cyclic AMP: pivotal role of M boxes (GTCATGTGCT) and of microphthalmia. *Mol. Cell. Biol.,* **1998,** *18*(2), 694-702.
[http://dx.doi.org/10.1128/MCB.18.2.694] [PMID: 9447965]

[46]   Rönnstrand, L. Signal transduction *via* the stem cell factor receptor/c-Kit. *Cell. Mol. Life Sci.,* **2004,** *61*(19-20), 2535-2548.
[http://dx.doi.org/10.1007/s00018-004-4189-6] [PMID: 15526160]

[47]   Halaban, R.; Langdon, R.; Birchall, N.; Cuono, C.; Baird, A.; Scott, G.; Moellmann, G.; McGuire, J. Basic fibroblast growth factor from human keratinocytes is a natural mitogen for melanocytes. *J. Cell Biol.,* **1988,** *107*(4), 1611-1619.
[http://dx.doi.org/10.1083/jcb.107.4.1611] [PMID: 2459134]

[48]   Puri, N.; van der Weel, M.B.; de Wit, F.S.; Asghar, S.S.; Das, P.K.; Ramaiah, A.; Westerhof, W. Basic fibroblast growth factor promotes melanin synthesis by melanocytes. *Arch. Dermatol. Res.,* **1996,** *288*(10), 633-635.
[http://dx.doi.org/10.1007/BF02505269] [PMID: 8919049]

[49]   Dong, L.; Li, Y.; Cao, J.; Liu, F.; Pier, E.; Chen, J.; Xu, Z.; Chen, C.; Wang, R.A.; Cui, R. FGF2 regulates melanocytes viability through the STAT3-transactivated PAX3 transcription. *Cell Death Differ.,* **2012,** *19*(4), 616-622.
[http://dx.doi.org/10.1038/cdd.2011.132] [PMID: 21997191]

[50]   Matsumoto, K.; Tajima, H.; Nakamura, T. Hepatocyte growth factor is a potent stimulator of human melanocyte DNA synthesis and growth. *Biochem. Biophys. Res. Commun.,* **1991,** *176*(1), 45-51.
[http://dx.doi.org/10.1016/0006-291X(91)90887-D] [PMID: 1708252]

[51]   Halaban, R.; Tyrrell, L.; Longley, J.; Yarden, Y.; Rubin, J. Pigmentation and proliferation of human melanocytes and the effects of melanocyte-stimulating hormone and ultraviolet B light. *Ann. N. Y. Acad. Sci.,* **1993,** *680,* 290-301.
[http://dx.doi.org/10.1111/j.1749-6632.1993.tb19691.x] [PMID: 7685575]

[52]   Hirobe, T. Role of keratinocyte-derived factors involved in regulating the proliferation and differentiation of mammalian epidermal melanocytes. *Pigment Cell Res.,* **2005,** *18*(1), 2-12.
[http://dx.doi.org/10.1111/j.1600-0749.2004.00198.x] [PMID: 15649147]

[53]   Choi, W.; Wolber, R.; Gerwat, W.; Mann, T.; Batzer, J.; Smuda, C.; Liu, H.; Kolbe, L.; Hearing, V.J. The fibroblast-derived paracrine factor neuregulin-1 has a novel role in regulating the constitutive color and melanocyte function in human skin. *J. Cell Sci.,* **2010,** *123*(Pt 18), 3102-3111.
[http://dx.doi.org/10.1242/jcs.064774] [PMID: 20736300]

[54]   Park, H.Y.; Wu, C.; Yonemoto, L.; Murphy-Smith, M.; Wu, H.; Stachur, C.M.; Gilchrest, B.A. MITF mediates cAMP-induced protein kinase C-β expression in human melanocytes. *Biochem. J.,* **2006,** *395*(3), 571-578.
[http://dx.doi.org/10.1042/BJ20051388] [PMID: 16411896]

[55]   Singh, S.K.; Abbas, W.A.; Tobin, D.J. Bone morphogenetic proteins differentially regulate pigmentation in human skin cells. *J. Cell Sci.,* **2012,** *125*(Pt 18), 4306-4319.
[http://dx.doi.org/10.1242/jcs.102038] [PMID: 22641693]

[56]   Kushimoto, T.; Basrur, V.; Valencia, J.; Matsunaga, J.; Vieira, W.D.; Ferrans, V.J.; Muller, J.; Appella, E.; Hearing, V.J. A model for melanosome biogenesis based on the purification and analysis of early melanosomes. *Proc. Natl. Acad. Sci. USA,* **2001**, *98*(19), 10698-10703.
[http://dx.doi.org/10.1073/pnas.191184798] [PMID: 11526213]

[57]   Raposo, G.; Marks, M.S. Melanosomes--dark organelles enlighten endosomal membrane transport. *Nat. Rev. Mol. Cell Biol.,* **2007**, *8*(10), 786-797.
[http://dx.doi.org/10.1038/nrm2258] [PMID: 17878918]

[58]   Fowler, D.M.; Koulov, A.V.; Alory-Jost, C.; Marks, M.S.; Balch, W.E.; Kelly, J.W. Functional amyloid formation within mammalian tissue. *PLoS Biol.,* **2006**, *4*(1), e6.
[http://dx.doi.org/10.1371/journal.pbio.0040006] [PMID: 16300414]

[59]   Theos, A.C.; Berson, J.F.; Theos, S.C.; Herman, K.E.; Harper, D.C.; Tenza, D.; Sviderskaya, E.V.; Lamoreux, M.L.; Bennett, D.C.; Raposo, G.; Marks, M.S. Dual loss of ER export and endocytic signals with altered melanosome morphology in the silver mutation of Pmel17. *Mol. Biol. Cell,* **2006**, *17*(8), 3598-3612.
[http://dx.doi.org/10.1091/mbc.e06-01-0081] [PMID: 16760433]

[60]   Leonhardt, R.M.; Vigneron, N.; Rahner, C.; Cresswell, P. Proprotein convertases process Pmel17 during secretion. *J. Biol. Chem.,* **2011**, *286*(11), 9321-9337.
[http://dx.doi.org/10.1074/jbc.M110.168088] [PMID: 21247888]

[61]   Delevoye, C.; Giordano, F.; van Niel, G.; Raposo, G. Biogenesis of melanosomes - the chessboard of pigmentation. *Med. Sci. (Paris),* **2011**, *27*(2), 153-162.
[http://dx.doi.org/10.1051/medsci/2011272153] [PMID: 21382323]

[62]   Incerti, B.; Cortese, K.; Pizzigoni, A.; Surace, E.M.; Varani, S.; Coppola, M.; Jeffery, G.; Seeliger, M.; Jaissle, G.; Bennett, D.C.; Marigo, V.; Schiaffino, M.V.; Tacchetti, C.; Ballabio, A. Oa1 knock-out: new insights on the pathogenesis of ocular albinism type 1. *Hum. Mol. Genet.,* **2000**, *9*(19), 2781-2788.
[http://dx.doi.org/10.1093/hmg/9.19.2781] [PMID: 11092754]

[63]   Lopez, V.M.; Decatur, C.L.; Stamer, W.D.; Lynch, R.M.; McKay, B.S. L-DOPA is an endogenous ligand for OA1. *PLoS Biol.,* **2008**, *6*(9), e236.
[http://dx.doi.org/10.1371/journal.pbio.0060236] [PMID: 18828673]

[64]   Giordano, F.; Bonetti, C.; Surace, E.M.; Marigo, V.; Raposo, G. The ocular albinism type 1 (OA1) G-protein-coupled receptor functions with MART-1 at early stages of melanogenesis to control melanosome identity and composition. *Hum. Mol. Genet.,* **2009**, *18*(23), 4530-4545.
[http://dx.doi.org/10.1093/hmg/ddp415] [PMID: 19717472]

[65]   Sitaram, A.; Marks, M.S. Mechanisms of protein delivery to melanosomes in pigment cells. *Physiology (Bethesda),* **2012**, *27*(2), 85-99.
[http://dx.doi.org/10.1152/physiol.00043.2011] [PMID: 22505665]

[66]   Di Pietro, S.M.; Falcón-Pérez, J.M.; Tenza, D.; Setty, S.R.G.; Marks, M.S.; Raposo, G.; Dell'Angelica, E.C. BLOC-1 interacts with BLOC-2 and the AP-3 complex to facilitate protein trafficking on endosomes. *Mol. Biol. Cell,* **2006**, *17*(9), 4027-4038.
[http://dx.doi.org/10.1091/mbc.e06-05-0379] [PMID: 16837549]

[67]   Setty, S.R.; Tenza, D.; Truschel, S.T.; Chou, E.; Sviderskaya, E.V.; Theos, A.C.; Lamoreux, M.L.; Di Pietro, S.M.; Starcevic, M.; Bennett, D.C.; Dell'Angelica, E.C.; Raposo, G.; Marks, M.S. BLOC-1 is required for cargo-specific sorting from vacuolar early endosomes toward lysosome-related organelles. *Mol. Biol. Cell,* **2007**, *18*(3), 768-780.
[http://dx.doi.org/10.1091/mbc.e06-12-1066] [PMID: 17182842]

[68]   Scott, G.; Leopardi, S.; Printup, S.; Madden, B.C. Filopodia are conduits for melanosome transfer to keratinocytes. *J. Cell Sci.,* **2002**, *115*(Pt 7), 1441-1451.
[PMID: 11896192]

[69]   Singh, S.K.; Kurfurst, R.; Nizard, C.; Schnebert, S.; Perrier, E.; Tobin, D.J. Melanin transfer in human skin cells is mediated by filopodia--a model for homotypic and heterotypic lysosome-related organelle transfer. *FASEB J.,* **2010**, *24*(10), 3756-3769.
[http://dx.doi.org/10.1096/fj.10-159046] [PMID: 20501793]

[70]   Liakath-Ali, K.; Vancollie, V.E.; Sequeira, I.; Lelliott, C.J.; Watt, F.M. Myosin 10 is involved in murine pigmentation. *Exp. Dermatol.,* **2019**, *28*(4), 391-394.
[http://dx.doi.org/10.1111/exd.13528] [PMID: 29509981]

[71]   Seiberg, M.; Paine, C.; Sharlow, E.; Andrade-Gordon, P.; Costanzo, M.; Eisinger, M.; Shapiro, S.S. The protease-activated receptor 2 regulates pigmentation *via* keratinocyte-melanocyte interactions. *Exp. Cell Res.,* **2000**, *254*(1), 25-32.
[http://dx.doi.org/10.1006/excr.1999.4692] [PMID: 10623462]

[72]   Scott, G.; Deng, A.; Rodriguez-Burford, C.; Seiberg, M.; Han, R.; Babiarz, L.; Grizzle, W.; Bell, W.; Pentland, A. Protease-activated receptor 2, a receptor involved in melanosome transfer, is upregulated in human skin by ultraviolet irradiation. *J. Invest. Dermatol.,* **2001**, *117*(6), 1412-1420.
[http://dx.doi.org/10.1046/j.0022-202x.2001.01575.x] [PMID: 11886502]

[73]   Sharlow, E.R.; Paine, C.S.; Babiarz, L.; Eisinger, M.; Shapiro, S.; Seiberg, M. The protease-activated receptor-2 upregulates keratinocyte phagocytosis. *J. Cell Sci.,* **2000**, *113*(Pt 17), 3093-3101.
[PMID: 10934047]

[74]   Scott, G.; Leopardi, S.; Parker, L.; Babiarz, L.; Seiberg, M.; Han, R. The proteinase-activated receptor-2 mediates phagocytosis in a Rho-dependent manner in human keratinocytes. *J. Invest. Dermatol.,* **2003**, *121*(3), 529-541.
[http://dx.doi.org/10.1046/j.1523-1747.2003.12427.x] [PMID: 12925212]

[75]   Cui, R.; Widlund, H.R.; Feige, E.; Lin, J.Y.; Wilensky, D.L.; Igras, V.E.; D'Orazio, J.; Fung, C.Y.; Schanbacher, C.F.; Granter, S.R.; Fisher, D.E. Central role of p53 in the suntan response and pathologic hyperpigmentation. *Cell,* **2007**, *128*(5), 853-864.
[http://dx.doi.org/10.1016/j.cell.2006.12.045] [PMID: 17350573]

[76]   Miyamura, Y.; Coelho, S.G.; Wolber, R.; Miller, S.A.; Wakamatsu, K.; Zmudzka, B.Z.; Ito, S.; Smuda, C.; Passeron, T.; Choi, W.; Batzer, J.; Yamaguchi, Y.; Beer, J.Z.; Hearing, V.J. Regulation of human skin pigmentation and responses to ultraviolet radiation. *Pigment Cell Res.,* **2007**, *20*(1), 2-13.
[http://dx.doi.org/10.1111/j.1600-0749.2006.00358.x] [PMID: 17250543]

[77]   Yamaguchi, Y.; Brenner, M.; Hearing, V.J. The regulation of skin pigmentation. *J. Biol. Chem.,* **2007**, *282*(38), 27557-27561.
[http://dx.doi.org/10.1074/jbc.R700026200] [PMID: 17635904]

[78]   Seiberg, M. Keratinocyte-melanocyte interactions during melanosome transfer. *Pigment Cell Res.,* **2001**, *14*(4), 236-242.
[http://dx.doi.org/10.1034/j.1600-0749.2001.140402.x] [PMID: 11549105]

[79]   Imokawa, G.; Yada, Y.; Miyagishi, M. Endothelins secreted from human keratinocytes are intrinsic mitogens for human melanocytes. *J. Biol. Chem.,* **1992**, *267*(34), 24675-24680.
[PMID: 1280264]

[80]   Yaar, M.; Grossman, K.; Eller, M.; Gilchrest, B.A. Evidence for nerve growth factor-mediated paracrine effects in human epidermis. *J. Cell Biol.,* **1991**, *115*(3), 821-828.
[http://dx.doi.org/10.1083/jcb.115.3.821] [PMID: 1655813]

[81]   Singh, S.K.; Baker, R.; Sikkink, S.K.; Nizard, C.; Schnebert, S.; Kurfurst, R.; Tobin, D.J. E-cadherin mediates ultraviolet radiation- and calcium-induced melanin transfer in human skin cells. *Exp. Dermatol.,* **2017**, *26*(11), 1125-1133.
[http://dx.doi.org/10.1111/exd.13395] [PMID: 28636748]

[82]   Starner, R.J.; McClelland, L.; Abdel-Malek, Z.; Fricke, A.; Scott, G. PGE(2) is a UVR-inducible autocrine factor for human melanocytes that stimulates tyrosinase activation. *Exp. Dermatol.,* **2010**,

19(7), 682-684.
[http://dx.doi.org/10.1111/j.1600-0625.2010.01074.x] [PMID: 20500768]

[83] Wicks, N.L.; Chan, J.W.; Najera, J.A.; Ciriello, J.M.; Oancea, E. UVA phototransduction drives early melanin synthesis in human melanocytes. *Curr. Biol.,* **2011**, *21*(22), 1906-1911.
[http://dx.doi.org/10.1016/j.cub.2011.09.047] [PMID: 22055294]

[84] Schecter, A.; Birnbaum, L.; Ryan, J.J.; Constable, J.D. Dioxins: an overview. *Environ. Res.,* **2006**, *101*(3), 419-428.
[http://dx.doi.org/10.1016/j.envres.2005.12.003] [PMID: 16445906]

[85] Nebert, D.W.; Dalton, T.P. The role of cytochrome P450 enzymes in endogenous signalling pathways and environmental carcinogenesis. *Nat. Rev. Cancer,* **2006**, *6*(12), 947-960.
[http://dx.doi.org/10.1038/nrc2015] [PMID: 17128211]

[86] Kawajiri, K.; Fujii-Kuriyama, Y. Cytochrome P450 gene regulation and physiological functions mediated by the aryl hydrocarbon receptor. *Arch. Biochem. Biophys.,* **2007**, *464*(2), 207-212.
[http://dx.doi.org/10.1016/j.abb.2007.03.038] [PMID: 17481570]

[87] Luecke, S.; Backlund, M.; Jux, B.; Esser, C.; Krutmann, J.; Rannug, A. The aryl hydrocarbon receptor (AHR), a novel regulator of human melanogenesis. *Pigment Cell Melanoma Res.,* **2010**, *23*(6), 828-833.
[http://dx.doi.org/10.1111/j.1755-148X.2010.00762.x] [PMID: 20973933]

[88] Shin, J.M.; Kim, M.Y.; Sohn, K.C.; Jung, S.Y.; Lee, H.E.; Lim, J.W.; Kim, S.; Lee, Y.H.; Im, M.; Seo, Y.J.; Kim, C.D.; Lee, J.H.; Lee, Y.; Yoon, T.J. Nrf2 negatively regulates melanogenesis by modulating PI3K/Akt signaling. *PLoS One,* **2014**, *9*(4), e96035.
[http://dx.doi.org/10.1371/journal.pone.0096035] [PMID: 24763530]

[89] Natale, C.A.; Duperret, E.K.; Zhang, J.; Sadeghi, R.; Dahal, A.; O'Brien, K.T.; Cookson, R.; Winkler, J.D.; Ridky, T.W. Sex steroids regulate skin pigmentation through nonclassical membrane-bound receptors. *eLife,* **2016**, *5*, e15104.
[http://dx.doi.org/10.7554/eLife.15104] [PMID: 27115344]

CHAPTER 4

Alteration in Melanogenesis: Pigmentary Disorders and their Etiopathogenesis

Abstract: Skin pigmentation contributes predominantly to the health and quality of life of human beings. Melanin imparts color to the skin, which is produced during the process of melanogenesis by the specialized cells, melanocytes. Many endogenous and exogenous factors released from epidermal and dermal components regulate constitutive skin pigmentation. The dysregulation of these factors followed by irregular production and distribution of melanin leads to the onset of pigmentary disorders such as hyperpigmentation or hypopigmentation. Pigmentation disorders include the entities that are characterized by a pathological change in melanocytes to produce melanin. Excess production of melanin leads to hyperpigmentary disorders and less or lack of melanin leads to hypopigmentary disorders. The present chapter is dedicated to the introduction and discussion of various pigmentary disorders with an overview of their etiologies and pathogenesis.

Keywords: Dysregulation, Hyperpigmentation, Hypopigmentation, Melanogenesis, Pigmentation.

1. INTRODUCTION

Color of the skin is due to the presence of melanin, a pigment produced by melanocytes, and normal pigmentation is dependent on the normal structure and function of these cells. Skin pigmentation is regulated by many factors for the proper development of melanocytes from their precursors. Development, maturation, trafficking of melanosomal components, melanin synthesis and further transport and distribution of melanosomes to the keratinocytes are also under the strict control of many factors secreted from melanocytes and keratinocytes respectively. Any defect affecting the complex process of skin pigmentation may result in the onset of pigmentary disorder, which may be either (a) hypopigmentary (b) or hyperpigmentary. Pathology of pigmentary disorders is related to the morphology of melanosome. It has been revealed that it is melanosome polymorphism such as variation in shape, size, fine-structural matrix, the degree of melanosomes maturation and the manner of melanin accumulation within it, which serves as a condition of the molecular pathology of various pig-

Sharique A. Ali & Naima Parveen

mentary disorders that could also be applied for diagnosis of these disorders [1, 2].

The hypopigmentary disorders are characterized by the less or lack of melanin produced by the melanocytes. These disorders were the most enigmatic issues since early days of human civilization. The first historical description of vitiligo was found during the period of Ausooryan (2200 BC) and has been discussed in *Tareekh-i-tibb-i-Iran* [3]. One of the earliest terms was "Kilas" in the Rig Veda, which was meant as similar to a white spotted deer [4]. Aulus Cornelius Celsus (25BC - 50 AD), a Latin medical author first introduced the term *"vitiligo"* in his book entitled *"De Medecina"* [5]. In 250 BC, Ptolemy II translated the Bible from Hebrew into Greek and in the Leviticus XIII (Old Testament), the word Zara'at was used for different skin conditions, which was translated as "lepros" (scales) that were misinterpreted later on as leprosy and other hypopigmented disorders, defined as unclean diseases [6, 7].

Accumulation of excess of melanin and its distribution leads to hyperpigmentary disorders. The problem of hyperpigmentation was also not considered normal from the ancient time. The hyperpigmentary conditions like melasma, birthmarks, and post inflammatory hyperpigmentation were relatively prevalent in all societies. However, in Atharva Veda (VII 8.1-8.II.10.1-B) mention of various *kshetriya* (hereditary and congenital) is available. In major Ayurveda texts, like *Charaka Samhita, Susruta Samhita, Astangahrdaya, Madhavanidan* and others, the very strong explanation of hyperpigmentary disorders is available [8, 9]. In the Greco-Arabic medicines, similar observations have been made. Various changes in skin color and their significance have been described in several sections of the Avicenna's *al-Qanun fi-al-tibb* (11th century AD) [10].

Vitiligo, albinism, Vogt-Koyanagi-Harada syndrome, idiopathic guttate hypo-melanosis, pityriasis alba are the diseases involving hypopigmentation. While post inflammatory hyperpigmentation, melasma, ephelide, solar lentigines, purigo pigmentosa, erythema dyschromicum perstans, lichen planus pigmentosus are the diseases involving hyperpigmentation. The present chapter describes the variations in skin pigmentation with a focus on pigmentation disorders and their etiopathogenesis.

2. HYPOPIGMENTATION DISEASES

2.1. Vitiligo

Vitiligo is an acquired, idiopathic disease which affects almost 0.2-2% of the world population. The disease is characterized by destroyed melanocytes that lead to patchy depigmentation. During the second century B.C., the term vitiligo was used for the first time by A.C. Celsus in his medical treatise *De medicina* [4, 11]. The term vitiligo comes from the latin word *vitium* which means defect or blemish. Vitiligo patients have many amelanotic, white or milky white patches or macules on their body. Usually, vitiligo patches are round and oval in shape. Vitiligo alters the quality of life of an affected person as it has psychosocial problems rather than clinical issues. Vitiligo is not a contagious and life threatening disease [12, 13].

Vitiligo can be classified into two major forms: segmental vitiligo and non segmental vitiligo. Non segmental vitiligo is characterized by depigmented macules, vary in size ranging from few to many centimetres in diameter. It comprises of different forms or types including acrofacial, universal, mucosal, and mixed vitiligo. Segmental vitiligo is characterized by a rapid progression of macule, but depigmentation spreads within the segment. Over a period of 6-24 months, extension of macules occurs. It usually has earlier age of onset than non segmental vitiligo. It can also be classified into three forms: Unisegmented, when only one segment is affected; Bisegmental, when two segments are affected; plurisegmental, in which more than two segments are affected [14, 15].

2.1.1. Pathogenesis of Vitiligo

Several theories have been proposed for explaining the pathogenesis of vitiligo:

2.1.1.1. Genetic Hypothesis

Most human diseases result from an interaction between genetic variants and environmental factors, and to establish the actual contribution of genetic factors is the first step of genetic studies that evaluate complex diseases. Epidemiological studies based on genetics concluded that vitiligo can be considered as a genetic disease because: (i) the disease varies in symptom rigorousness and the age of onset, which hampers the definition of the appropriate phenotype and the selection of the most favourable study population; the onset of disease in the early age was associated with familial occurrence of generalized vitiligo [16, 17]. Early onset vitiligo is also associated with more severe disease; (ii) the etiological mechanisms of the disease can vary; vitiligo's etiopathogenesis has not yet been fully understood, and various theories have been proposed; (iii) More often, the complex genetic diseases are oligogenic or even polygenic and each gene takes part to a fraction of the overall relative risk.

The involvement of genetic factors in the susceptibility to vitiligo became evident in familial studies, which demonstrated that vitiligo segregates with a complex standard of multifactorial and polygenic inheritance. Ando *et al.* [18], during one of their experiments found that there was a significant interaction between HLA-B46 and familial non segmental vitiligo in 131 Japanese patients, whereas HLA-A31 and CW4 were found in nonfamilial patients.

Additionally, around 50 candidate genes have already been investigated in association studies for susceptibility to vitiligo. However, only a few genes present a clear association with vitiligo. On the one hand, there are non-HLA genes, including DDR1, XBP1, NLRP1, PTPN22 and COMT; on the other hand, there are HLA-associated genes, including HLA-A2, HLA-DR4 and HLA-DR7 alleles [19]. Hence, genetic factors probably play an essential role in the pathogenesis of vitiligo, but the exact genetic defects remain to be identified.

2.1.1.2. Autoimmune Hypothesis

Autoimmune hypothesis is one of the most significant and popular hypotheses. This hypothesis suggests that abnormality of the immune system results in destruction of melanocytes. Substantial new data implicate immune mechanisms in the pathogenesis of vitiligo and indicate that vitiligo may share common linkages with other autoimmune diseases (thyroid disorders, juvenile diabetes mellitus, and Addison's disease, pernicious anaemia) [16, 20].

Vitiligo is accompanied by abnormal cellular and humoral immunity. Elevated levels of serum circulating autoantibodies particularly of the IgG class have been observed in 5-10% of vitiligo patients. However, the function of antimelanocyte antibodies in vitiligo pathogenesis remains unsure and it has been suggested that their presence may be secondary to melanocyte and keratinocyte damages [21, 22].

In the margins of lesional and normal pigmented skin of patients with active vitiligo or inflammatory vitiligo, a mild mononuclear cell infiltrate can be observed. Immuno histochemical studies indicated that it is T cells that are abundant in these infiltrates; T cells may therefore play a major role in the destruction of melanocytes. More recently, an *in vitro* study showed that cytotoxic T lymphocytes infiltrated in common vitiligo perilesional area destroyed neighbouring melanocytes [23, 24]. Different abnormalities in peripheral blood mononuclear cells have also been described. Levels of natural killer cells, CD4+ and CD8+ have been reported to be normal, increased or decreased. Various factors are known to influence these parameters and they are not standardized in any of the studies conducted [25] (Fig. **1**).

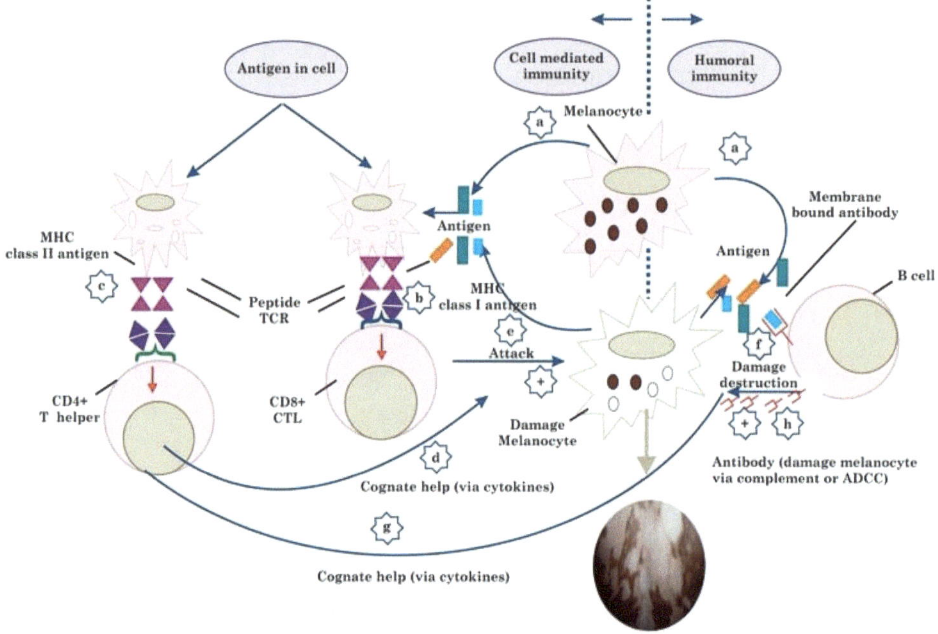

Fig. (1). Pathway of vitiligo progression (autoimmune): There are two major proposed autoimmune mechanisms of vitiligo pathogenesis; one antibody (humoral) based and another T-cell (cellular) based. The most direct evidence to support autoimmunity hypothesis is that the majority of patients with vitiligo have circulating antibodies to surface and cytoplasmic melanocytes antigens. The increase in the level of antibodies and/or cytotoxic T-cells close to damaged melanocytes suggested that the mode of action cells takes against melanocytes for vitiligo progression is apoptosis induction directly against melanocytes or antibody (Ig) generated complement system and T-cell mediated.

2.1.1.3. Neural Hypothesis

The neural hypothesis was first suggested by Lerner [26], where it was reported that there is a presence of certain neurochemical mediators that are cytotoxic to melanocytes which are secreted from nearby nerve endings. This theory is supported by the following clinical interpretations:

1. The existence of the localized form of vitiligo that seems to be limited to one segment of the body. This 'segemental' vitiligo is approximately non dermatomal but normally affects portions of multiple dermatomes. It is also assumed that segmental vitiligo does not act in response to classical vitiligo therapies, such as PUVA, but to agents that modulate neural function.
2. The onset of vitiligo is reported after a severe emotional stress. The mechanism by which stress results into depigmentation is not clear.
3. It is also reported that vitiligo occurs in patients with neurological disorders, in

a child with viral encephalitis, in multiple sclerosis and in a patient with peripheral nerve injury [27].

2.1.1.4. Autocytotoxic Hypothesis

This theory proposed that the precursors of melanogenesis are toxic to melanocytes. Melanocytes have an intracellular protective meachnism in order to eliminate toxic melanin precursors (*e.g.* dopa, dopachrome and 5,6-dihydroxyindole) and free radicals. In vitiligo, there may be some hindrance of this mechanism, resulting in an accumulation of indoles and free radicals that destruct melanocytes [28].

2.1.1.5. Growth Factor Defect Hypothesis

In 1987, Puri *et al.* [29], postulated that the defective growth of melanocyte originated from non lesional and peri lesional skin. Surprisingly, the investigators observed that the defects were corrected partially by *in vitro* supplementation of fetal lung fibroblast derived growth factors. Their finding suggests that growth defects play an essential role in pathogenesis of vitiligo. Further studies are required to evaluate the use of growth factors, as a part of repigmentation therapy in vitiligo.

2.1.1.6. Adhesion Defect Theory

Gauthier *et al.* [30] proposed that non segmental vitiligo might be caused by a chronic detachment of melanocytes stimulated by trauma, mainly a mechanical rubbing of healthy skin. This concept is called as "melanocytorrhagy theory". Furthermore, Gauthier *et al.* hypothesized that an autoimmune activation could be provoked by dendritic cells or memory T cells detecting auto-antigens during melanocytorrhagy through the epidermis basal layer [31].

2.1.1.7. Convergence Theory

It has been suggested that a combined theory rather than a separate theory is more suitable in the etiology. Furthermore, the studies that the patients exhibit a variety of clinical forms and various histories of onset of disease make us believe that the etiology of vitiligo may vary among individuals. This theory suggests that stress, genetic factors, autoimmunity, accumulation of toxic compounds, infections, mutation, varied cellular environment and impaired melanocyte migration and proliferation can all contribute to the phenomenon of vitiligo [32].

2.2. Albinism

Albinism is characterized by less or no pigmentation in the skin, hairs and eyes due to the inherited deficiency of enzyme tyrosinase, which is the key enzyme of melanogenesis. The worldwide prevalence of albinism is approximately one among the twenty thousand individuals. It can be seen in all ethnic groups but may vary among the different forms and featured to different gene mutations. Usually 11 types exhibiting autosomal recessive transmission and the disease severity is different in different types. The most severe form is Type 1 albinism (oculocutaneous albinism), in which tyrosinase is totally absent because coding TYR gene is defective. Person with type 1 albinism cannot tan even though he or she can go out in sun and having complete white skin and hairs [33]. In Type II albinism tyrosinase activity is partial and can synthesize melanin but at very low rate. Patients with type II albinism have cream or light brown hairs and grey or light brown eyes [34]. In clinical practice, loss of iris pigmentation, loss of hearing, decreased retinal pigment in the epithelium, loss of visual acuity, photophobia *etc.* can also be seen in albinism. Despite of defective pigmentation, albinism patients exhibit normal development in terms of intelligence and fertility. They are advised to do skin examination regularly so that skin cancer can be diagnosed and treated at an early stage [35].

2.3. Idiopathic Guttate Hypomelanosis (IGH)

It is a leucodermic dermatosis, commonly seen in middle or old aged women. Pathogenesis of IGH includes actinic injury triggered by photoaging and UV light. Macules are usually seen on the external surfaces of the patient but are also observed on abdomen and chest. Macules are 2-10 mm in size with sharp margins. Topical tacrolimus, 88% phenol and pimecrolimus, ablated or fractionated carbondioxide laser are the treatment modalities used to cure IGH [36].

2.4. Pityriasis Alba

Pityriasis alba (PA) is the most common hypopigmentary disorder which occurs in children of age 6-16 years. It is a chronic disease characterized by scattered hypopigmented macules on the skin of the individual. It affects almost 1% of the total population and 9% of the pediatric population. Irregular and undefined hypopigmented lesions on the face, trunk, and arms are generally seen in clinical practise. These macules or lesions are 0.5 to 6 cm in size. Dry skin, exposure to sun and light are implicated in pathogenesis. Treatment can be done by sun protector, moisturizers, corticosteroid and antiseptics. Topical application of immunosuppressive agents such as tacrolimus and pimecrolimus was found to be perfect for the treatment of PA [37, 38]. Moreno-Cruz *et al.* [37] on comparing the results of calcipotriol and tacrolimus in PA, found that both are similarly effective on PA. But, they have been reported that calcipotriol represents the better alternative therapeutic as it lacks the long term side effects of immunosuppresives.

2.5. Vogt-Koyanagi-Harada Syndrome

Vogt-Koyanagi- Harada syndrome is very rare autoimmune disease which occurs in dark skinned young or old women aged 20-50 years. General cause of the disease is uncertain but it is assumed that genetic factors may involve. The classical appearance of the patient includes hypoacusia, vitiligo, poliosis with meningitis. The person taking high dose of systemic steroids is found to be more rapidly attacked by the disease [39].

3. HYPERPIGMENTATION DISORDERS

3.1. Post Inflammatory Hyperpigmentation

The most common dermatoses seen in African American patients other than vitiligo were post inflammatory hyper pigmentation (PIH). Physical examination of PIH is small to large hyper pigmented macules of various sizes in any distribution. There are various causes of PIH including infections such as dermatophytoses, allergic reactions such as those from insect bites or contact dermatitis, medication or drug reaction, and cutanoeus injury from burns, irritants or cosmetic therapies [40]. But Taylor *et al.* [41] have demonstrated *Acne vulgaris* as the major cause of PIH. From their study they have evaluated that 65.5% of African American, 52.7% of Hispanic and 47.4% of Asian patients developed acne induced PIH. PIH occur in both epidermis and dermis of the skin. In epidermal PIH, melanin production and its transfer to keratinocytes increases. In dermal PIH, a damaged basement membrane allows melanin to enter dermis that is phagocytosed by dermal macrophages [42].

3.2. Melasma

Melasma, a common and well described form of hyper pigmentation affecting millions of people worldwide and around 90% of those are females. It affects women with darker skin types including Fitzpatrick skin phototypes III and IV. Melasma is also called as chloasma or the mask of pregnancy because the condition is often associated with pregnant women. There is no exact etiology of melasma but multiple factors like ultraviolet radiation, genetic predisposition, hormonal changes and inflammation have been involved. Clinically they are light to dark brown macules with irregular margins commonly distributed symmetrically on the malar, mandubuar and centrofacial regions and can also be seen on the forearms [43].

Melasma can be differentiated into dermal, epidermal, mixed and interdeterminate types. Pigment is brown and borders are well defined in epidermal type whereas in dermal type pigment is grey brown and borders are poorly defined. Mixed type melasma occurs when there is increase in melanin in both epidermis and dermis but interdeterminate type of melasma is not easy to classify even with the use of Wood's light [44]. A recent cross sectional multicentric study conducted by Sarkar *et al.* [45] has found that melasma mostly occured in females of intermediate skin phototypes in comparison to males.

3.3. Ephelides and Solar Lentigines

Solar lentigines have been reported in white subjects including African-American and American- Indians. It is more likely to occur in individuals of skin type I and III. The main cause of lentigines is the local propagation of basal melanocytes and a subsequent increase in melanisation. They occur on sun exposed areas predominantly on face, dorsal side of hands and forearms, upper back and chest [46]. Ephelides or freckles are different from solar lentigines and are caused by increase in photoinduced melanogenesis. But some of the ephelides represent as a subtype of solar lentigo. Like lentigines, it also occurs on sun exposed area of the body particularly on dorsal side of the hands or trunk and face. They are 1-3 mm hyper pigmented macules which are round, oval, or irregular in shape [47]. Ephelides are generally benign and show no susceptibility for malignant transformation [48].

3.4. Lichen Planus Pigmentosus

Kanwar *et al.* [49] have studied 124 Indian patients with Lichen planus pigmentosus. They described it as unusual variant of lichen planus common in individual with skin type III and IV. It affects young to middle aged individuals usually those from India, America, and the Middle East. Physical examination of the disease revealed presence of oval or irregular grey-brown to brown patches or macules with generally diffused and symmetrical pattern. They occur on sunexposed areas including face, neck and forearms. The etiology of the disease is not clear, but exposure to ultraviolet light and immunological mechanisms associated with cellular immunity appears to be concerned [50]. The coexistence of linear and inversus variants of lichen planus pigmentosus was also observed, which was of rare occurrence [51].

3.5. Erythema Dyschromicum Perstans (EDP)

EDP is characterized by slowly progressive, asymptomatic ash colored lesions hence also called as ashy dermatosis. Some workers also consider it as antithesis of lichen planus pigmentosus. The condition is still controversial due to clinical and histopathological chracteristics of the disease. The cause of the disease is uncertain and the disease is more common in dark skinned individuals. Clinically, grey, grey-brown or grey-blue lesions can be seen on face, trunk, neck and arms. Vacuoles in the basal layer and varying degree of lichenoid lymphocytic infiltration and colloid bodies are observed during pathological diagnosis of the disease. Treatment includes chemical peeling, topical and systemic steroids but found to be ineffective. Clofazimine, dapsone and griseofulvin are the drugs which have been shown effective somehow [52, 53].

3.6. Prurigo Pigmentosa (PP)

Prurigo pigmentosa is an inflammatory dermatosis disease characterized by symmetric and itchy erythematous urticarial macules on the neck and trunk accompanied by irregular pigmentation. Some studies have reported that it may be associated with certain other conditions and diseases including pregnancy, diabetes mellitus, diet, ketonemia, weight gain, menstruation. Through pathological investigation, hyperplasia and parakeratosis in the epidermis and hyperpigmentation with melanophages in the upper dermis were observed. Minocycline in an oral dose of 100 mg/day is used for its treatment. Dapson, doxycycline, potassium iodide and some antibiotics from the macrolide groups have also found effective [54, 55].

3.7. Maturational Dyschromia

Maturational dyschromia is characterized as diffused hyperpigmentation, which occurs on the cheekbones and lateral forehead. It is described as general uneven skin tone, complaint by more than one third of the dark women. It may be misdiagnosed as post inflammatory hyperpigmentaion (PIH), or EDP. Use of sunscreen, skin lightening agents, and antioxidants are the treatment options for maturational dyschromia. Microdermabrasion and chemical peeling have also been reported as potentially effective [56].

3.8. Riehl Melanosis

Riehl melanosis is a pigmented contact dermatitis that is characterized by brown or grey colored secondary melanin deposit. The disease is initiated as mild erythema followed by diffuse to reticulate hyperpigmented macules. Diagnosis can be done by close patch testing to standard series and cosmetic series. Sometimes photopatch can also be considered [57]. A very rarely occurred variant of Reihl melanosis called erythrose peribuccale pigmentaire de Brocq is caused by photodynamic substances in cosmetic products. It is described as diffuse, symmetric hyperpigmentary lesions around the mouth and extended to the forehead. Use of skin lightening agents, chemical peels, sun protective measures, and avoidance of suspected allergens completely are the various treatments that can be done for Reihl melanosis [44].

3.9. Acanthosis Nigricans

Acanthosis nigricans is characterized by hyperpigmented and velvety macules in a symmetric distribution, and it is more common in Hispanic and dark people. It occurs in almost any location including face, posterior neck, intertriginous areas of the axilla. The disease is associated with insulin resistance and obesity. There is no treatment found for acanthosis nigricans but certain topical combinations have tried including keratolytics, a combination of topical tretinoin 0.05% and ammonium lactate 12% cream and triple combination depigmenting cream, a combination of tretinoin 0.05%, hydroquinone 4%, fluocinolone acetonide 0.01%. Salicylic acid, urea, calcipotriol and podophyllin have also been reported to use for acanthosis nigricans [58, 59].

3.10. Naevus of Ota

The disease is characterized by blue grey plaques with diamter ranging from pin head size to several millimetres. Most commonly appears on periorbital area, forehead, malar area, earlobe, nose, conjunctivae, retroauricular regions *etc.* Naevus of Ota generally occurred in all skin types but predominantly has been documented in dark people, especially Asians. The macules or plaques occur during infancy, with the majority appearing at birth and also around puberty. Onset of the disease was found between 1 and 11 years of age but after the age of 20, it is unusual. Treatment with Q- switched ruby, Nd-YAG lasers have been reported effective for Naevus of Ota [60, 61].

3.11. Exogeneous Ochronosis

It is a rare disease characterized by blue- black hyperpigmented macules caused by the deposition of polymerized homogentisic acid in collagen containing structures. The most common sites of involvement are face, back, neck, and other extensor surfaces. Exogeneous ochronosis is clinically similar to endogeneous ochronosis, also called as alkaptonuria which is inherited disorder but exogeneous ochronosis exhibits no systemic effects and not an inherited disorder [62]. It is caused by the continuous use of products containing resorcinol, hydroquinone, picric acid and heavy metals like mercury. It is more prevalent in African people [63]. Histological confirmation is required in exogeneous ochronosis as it is easily be confused with post inflammatory hyperpigmentation, melasma, contact dermatitis. Treatment of exogeneous ochronosis includes dermabrasion, chemical peel, Q-switched laser *etc.* [64]. The above discussed disorders are systematically written in Table **1** along with their etiology.

Table 1. Forms of pigmentation disorders with etiology.

Pigmentation Disorder	Location	Etiology	Description
Hypopigmentation Disorders			
Vitiligo	Face, hands, forearms, neck, genitalia, body folds, periorificial; lip-tip pattern	Unknown, possibly immune-mediated	Hypo and amelanotic macules and patches; sharply defined; 5 to 10 cm either isolated or coalescent
Idiopathic guttate hypomelanosis	external surfaces but are also observed on abdomen and chest	Actinic injury triggered by photoaging and UV light.	Macules are 2-10 mm in size with sharp margins
Pityriasis alba	Face, head, neck, forearms	Possible association with atopic dermatitis aggravated by sunlight exposure	Hypopigmented, irregular patches; fine scale; itchy
Albinism (Type I and type II)	Complete body Skin, hairs	Inherited deficiency of enzyme tyrosinase	Complete amelanotic skin and hairs in type I and cream or light brown hairs and grey or light brown eyes in type II
Hyperpigmentation disorders			
Post inflammatory hyperpigmentation	Previous sites of injury or inflammation	Trauma, inflammation	Irregular, darkly pigmented macules/patches
Solar lentigines	Face, hands, forearms, chest, back, shins	Acute or chronic ultraviolet exposure	1- to 3-cm well circumscribed macules; light yellow to dark brown, variegated

(Table 1) cont.....

Pigmentation Disorder	Location	Etiology	Description
Ephelides	Face, neck, chest, arms, legs	Childhood onset after sun exposure in susceptible individuals (skin types I or II)	2 to 3 mm sharply defined macules, tan to light brown
Melasma	Face (centrofacial 63%, malar 21%, mandibular 16%) or forearms	Pregnancy, oral contraceptives, phenytoin (Dilantin), idiopathic	Pigmented, well-defined macules; light brown, brown, or gray

CONCLUSION

The present chapter discusses variation in pigmentation in the form of hypo and hyperpigmentation disorders. This is a disease group that occupies a significant place among diseases of the skin and that is predominantly worrying in cosmetic terms. Increasing dermatologists and other physicians experience and knowledge regarding differential diagnosis and treatment will assist correct management of these pigmentation disorders at a great extent.

REFERENCES

[1]   Rose, P.T. Pigmentary disorders. *Med. Clin. North Am.,* **2009**, *93*(6), 1225-1239.
[http://dx.doi.org/10.1016/j.mcna.2009.08.005] [PMID: 19932328]

[2]   Bastonini, E.; Kovacs, D.; Picardo, M. Skin pigmentation and pigmentary disorders: focus on epidermal/dermal cross-talk. *Ann. Dermatol.,* **2016**, *28*(3), 279-289.
[http://dx.doi.org/10.5021/ad.2016.28.3.279] [PMID: 27274625]

[3]   Prasad, P.V.; Bhatnagar, V.K. Medico-historical study of "Kilasa" (vitiligo/leucoderma) a common skin disorder. *Bull. Indian Inst. Hist. Med. Hyderabad,* **2003**, *33*(2), 113-127.
[PMID: 17154114]

[4]   Nair, B.K. Vitiligo--a retrospect. *Int. J. Dermatol.,* **1978**, *17*(9), 755-757.
[http://dx.doi.org/10.1111/ijd.1978.17.9.755] [PMID: 365814]

[5]   Verbov, J. Celsus and his contributions to Dermatology. *Int. J. Dermatol.,* **1978**, *17*(6), 521-523.
[http://dx.doi.org/10.1111/j.1365-4362.1978.tb06191.x] [PMID: 355170]

[6]   Goldman, L.; Moraites, R.S.; Kitzmiller, K.W. White spots in biblical times. A background for the dermatologist for participation in discussions of current revisions of the bible. *Arch. Dermatol.,* **1966**, *93*(6), 744-753.
[http://dx.doi.org/10.1001/archderm.1966.01600240110023] [PMID: 5326716]

[7]   Freilich, A.R. Tzaraat--"biblical leprosy". *J. Am. Acad. Dermatol.,* **1982**, *6*(1), 131-134.
[http://dx.doi.org/10.1016/S0190-9622(82)70010-6] [PMID: 7045170]

[8]   Sen, D.N.; Sen, U.N. *Sarira Sthanam*; Charaka Samhita: Calcutta, **1897**, verse 14, .

[9]   Sen, S.K.K.; Bhattacharya, S.S. Sarangdhara: Chikitsa Samgraha. Kolkata: Dipayan. *Purvakhanda,* **1998**, *VII*, 84-92.

[10]   Gruner, O.C. *A treatise on the Canon of the Medicine of Avicenna*; AMS Press Inc. Aphorism 221 and 795: New York, **1973**.

[11]   Gauthier, Y.; Benzekri, L. Historical aspects. In: *Vitiligo*; Picardo, M.; Taïeb, A., Eds.; Springer Verlag: Heidelberg, **2010**; pp. 3-9.
[http://dx.doi.org/10.1007/978-3-540-69361-1_1]

[12]   Koranne, R.V.; Sachdeva, K.G. Vitiligo. *Int. J. Dermatol.*, **1988**, *27*(10), 676-681.
[http://dx.doi.org/10.1111/j.1365-4362.1988.tb01260.x] [PMID: 3069756]

[13]   Sehgal, V.N.; Srivastava, G. Vitiligo: compendium of clinico-epidemiological features. *Indian J. Dermatol. Venereol. Leprol.*, **2007**, *73*(3), 149-156.
[http://dx.doi.org/10.4103/0378-6323.32708] [PMID: 17558045]

[14]   Koga, M.; Tango, T. Clinical features and course of type A and type B vitiligo. *Br. J. Dermatol.*, **1988**, *118*(2), 223-228.
[http://dx.doi.org/10.1111/j.1365-2133.1988.tb01778.x] [PMID: 3348967]

[15]   Ezzedine, K.; Lim, H.W.; Suzuki, T.; Katayama, I.; Hamzavi, I.; Lan, C.C.; Goh, B.K.; Anbar, T.; Silva de Castro, C.; Lee, A.Y.; Parsad, D.; van Geel, N.; Le Poole, I.C.; Oiso, N.; Benzekri, L.; Spritz, R.; Gauthier, Y.; Hann, S.K.; Picardo, M.; Taieb, A. Vitiligo Global Issue Consensus Conference Panelists. Revised classification/nomenclature of vitiligo and related issues: the Vitiligo Global Issues Consensus Conference. *Pigment Cell Melanoma Res.*, **2012**, *25*(3), E1-E13.
[http://dx.doi.org/10.1111/j.1755-148X.2012.00997.x] [PMID: 22417114]

[16]   Alkhateeb, A.; Fain, P.R.; Thody, A.; Bennett, D.C.; Spritz, R.A. Epidemiology of vitiligo and associated autoimmune diseases in Caucasian probands and their families. *Pigment Cell Res.*, **2003**, *16*(3), 208-214.
[http://dx.doi.org/10.1034/j.1600-0749.2003.00032.x] [PMID: 12753387]

[17]   Laberge, G.; Mailloux, C.M.; Gowan, K.; Holland, P.; Bennett, D.C.; Fain, P.R.; Spritz, R.A. Early disease onset and increased risk of other autoimmune diseases in familial generalized vitiligo. *Pigment Cell Res.*, **2005**, *18*(4), 300-305.
[http://dx.doi.org/10.1111/j.1600-0749.2005.00242.x] [PMID: 16029422]

[18]   Ando, I.; Chi, H.I.; Nakagawa, H.; Otsuka, F. Difference in clinical features and HLA antigens between familial and non-familial vitiligo of non-segmental type. *Br. J. Dermatol.*, **1993**, *129*(4), 408-410.
[http://dx.doi.org/10.1111/j.1365-2133.1993.tb03167.x] [PMID: 8217754]

[19]   Singh, A.; Sharma, P.; Kar, H.K.; Sharma, V.K.; Tembhre, M.K.; Gupta, S.; Laddha, N.C.; Dwivedi, M.; Begum, R.; Gokhale, R.S.; Rani, R. Indian Genome Variation Consortium. HLA alleles and amino-acid signatures of the peptide-binding pockets of HLA molecules in vitiligo. *J. Invest. Dermatol.*, **2012**, *132*(1), 124-134.
[http://dx.doi.org/10.1038/jid.2011.240] [PMID: 21833019]

[20]   Levandowski, C.B.; Mailloux, C.M.; Ferrara, T.M.; Gowan, K.; Ben, S.; Jin, Y.; McFann, K.K.; Holland, P.J.; Fain, P.R.; Dinarello, C.A.; Spritz, R.A. NLRP1 haplotypes associated with vitiligo and autoimmunity increase interleukin-1β processing *via* the NLRP1 inflammasome. *Proc. Natl. Acad. Sci. USA*, **2013**, *110*(8), 2952-2956.
[http://dx.doi.org/10.1073/pnas.1222808110] [PMID: 23382179]

[21]   Kemp, E.H.; Waterman, E.A.; Hawes, B.E.; O'Neill, K.; Gottumukkala, R.V.; Gawkrodger, D.J.; Weetman, A.P.; Watson, P.F. The melanin-concentrating hormone receptor 1, a novel target of autoantibody responses in vitiligo. *J. Clin. Invest.*, **2002**, *109*(7), 923-930.
[http://dx.doi.org/10.1172/JCI0214643] [PMID: 11927619]

[22]   Schallreuter, K.U.; Bahadoran, P.; Picardo, M.; Slominski, A.; Elassiuty, Y.E.; Kemp, E.H.; Giachino, C.; Liu, J.B.; Luiten, R.M.; Lambe, T.; Le Poole, I.C.; Dammak, I.; Onay, H.; Zmijewski, M.A.; Dell'Anna, M.L.; Zeegers, M.P.; Cornall, R.J.; Paus, R.; Ortonne, J.P.; Westerhof, W. Vitiligo pathogenesis: autoimmune disease, genetic defect, excessive reactive oxygen species, calcium imbalance, or what else? *Exp. Dermatol.*, **2008**, *17*(2), 139-140.
[http://dx.doi.org/10.1111/j.1600-0625.2007.00666.x] [PMID: 18205713]

[23]   van den Boorn, J.G.; Konijnenberg, D.; Dellemijn, T.A.; van der Veen, J.P.; Bos, J.D.; Melief, C.J.; Vyth-Dreese, F.A.; Luiten, R.M. Autoimmune destruction of skin melanocytes by perilesional T cells from vitiligo patients. *J. Invest. Dermatol.,* **2009**, *129*(9), 2220-2232.
        [http://dx.doi.org/10.1038/jid.2009.32] [PMID: 19242513]

[24]   Shen, C.; Gao, J.; Sheng, Y.; Dou, J.; Zhou, F.; Zheng, X.; Ko, R.; Tang, X.; Zhu, C.; Yin, X.; Sun, L.; Cui, Y.; Zhang, X. Genetic Susceptibility to Vitiligo: GWAS Approaches for Identifying Vitiligo Susceptibility Genes and Loci. *Front. Genet.,* **2016**, *7*, 3.
        [http://dx.doi.org/10.3389/fgene.2016.00003] [PMID: 26870082]

[25]   Zhou, L.; Li, K.; Shi, Y.L.; Hamzavi, I.; Gao, T.W.; Henderson, M.; Huggins, R.H.; Agbai, O.; Mahmoud, B.; Mi, X.; Lim, H.W.; Mi, Q.S. Systemic analyses of immunophenotypes of peripheral T cells in non-segmental vitiligo: implication of defective natural killer T cells. *Pigment Cell Melanoma Res.,* **2012**, *25*(5), 602-611.
        [http://dx.doi.org/10.1111/j.1755-148X.2012.01019.x] [PMID: 22591262]

[26]   Lerner, A.B. Vitiligo. *J. Invest. Dermatol.,* **1959**, *32*(2, Part 2), 285-310.
        [http://dx.doi.org/10.1038/jid.1959.49] [PMID: 13641799]

[27]   Poojary, S.; Minni, K. Genetics of Vitiligo: An Insight. *J. Pigment. Disord.,* **2015**, *2*, 178.
        [http://dx.doi.org/10.4172/2376-0427.1000178]

[28]   Boissy, R.E.; Manga, P. On the etiology of contact/occupational vitiligo. *Pigment Cell Res.,* **2004**, *17*(3), 208-214.
        [http://dx.doi.org/10.1111/j.1600-0749.2004.00130.x] [PMID: 15140065]

[29]   Puri, N.; Mojamdar, M.; Ramaiah, A. *In vitro* growth characteristics of melanocytes obtained from adult normal and vitiligo subjects. *J. Invest. Dermatol.,* **1987**, *88*(4), 434-438.
        [http://dx.doi.org/10.1111/1523-1747.ep12469795] [PMID: 3559270]

[30]   Gauthier, Y.; Cario Andre, M.; Taieb, A. A critical appraisal of vitiligo etiologic theories. Is melanocyte loss a melanocytorrhagy? *Pigment Cell Res,* **2003**, *16*, 322-332.

[31]   Gauthier, Y.; Cario-Andre, M.; Lepreux, S.; Pain, C.; Taïeb, A. Melanocyte detachment after skin friction in non lesional skin of patients with generalized vitiligo. *Br. J. Dermatol.,* **2003**, *148*, 95-101.
        [http://dx.doi.org/10.1046/j.1365-2133.2003.05024.x]

[32]   Le Poole, I.C.; Das, P.K.; van den Wijngaard, R.M.; Bos, J.D.; Westerhof, W. Review of the etiopathomechanism of vitiligo: a convergence theory. *Exp. Dermatol.,* **1993**, *2*(4), 145-153.
        [http://dx.doi.org/10.1111/j.1600-0625.1993.tb00023.x] [PMID: 8162332]

[33]   Simeonov, D.R.; Wang, X.; Wang, C.; Sergeev, Y.; Dolinska, M.; Bower, M.; Fischer, R.; Winer, D.; Dubrovsky, G.; Balog, J.Z.; Huizing, M.; Hart, R.; Zein, W.M.; Gahl, W.A.; Brooks, B.P.; Adams, D.R. DNA variations in oculocutaneous albinism: an updated mutation list and current outstanding issues in molecular diagnostics. *Hum. Mutat.,* **2013**, *34*(6), 827-835.
        [http://dx.doi.org/10.1002/humu.22315] [PMID: 23504663]

[34]   Dotta, L.; Parolini, S.; Prandini, A.; Tabellini, G.; Antolini, M.; Kingsmore, S.F.; Badolato, R. Clinical, laboratory and molecular signs of immunodeficiency in patients with partial oculo-cutaneous albinism. *Orphanet J. Rare Dis.,* **2013**, *8*, 168.
        [http://dx.doi.org/10.1186/1750-1172-8-168] [PMID: 24134793]

[35]   Grønskov, K.; Ek, J.; Brondum-Nielsen, K. Oculocutaneous albinism. *Orphanet J. Rare Dis.,* **2007**, *2*, 43.
        [http://dx.doi.org/10.1186/1750-1172-2-43] [PMID: 17980020]

[36]   Joshi, R. Skip areas of retained melanin: a clue to the histopathological diagnosis of idiopathic guttate hypomelanosis. *Indian J. Dermatol.,* **2014**, *59*(6), 571-574.
        [http://dx.doi.org/10.4103/0019-5154.143516] [PMID: 25484386]

[37]   Moreno-Cruz, B.; Torres-Álvarez, B.; Hernández-Blanco, D.; Castanedo-Cazares, J.P. Double-blind, placebo-controlled, randomized study comparing 0.0003% calcitriol with 0.1% tacrolimus ointments

for the treatment of endemic pityriasis alba. *Dermatol. Res. Pract.,* **2012**, *2012*, 303275.
[http://dx.doi.org/10.1155/2012/303275] [PMID: 22577371]

[38]   Carneiro, F.R.; Amaral, G.B.; Mendes, M.D.; Quaresma, J.A. Tissue immunostaining for factor XIIIa in dermal dendrocytes of pityriasis alba skin lesions. *An. Bras. Dermatol.,* **2014**, *89*(2), 245-248.
[http://dx.doi.org/10.1590/abd1806-4841.20142201] [PMID: 24770500]

[39]   Greco, A.; Fusconi, M.; Gallo, A.; Turchetta, R.; Marinelli, C.; Macri, G.F.; De Virgilio, A.; de Vincentiis, M. Vogt-Koyanagi-Harada syndrome. *Autoimmun. Rev.,* **2013**, *12*(11), 1033-1038.
[http://dx.doi.org/10.1016/j.autrev.2013.01.004] [PMID: 23567866]

[40]   Halder, R.M.; Grimes, P.E.; McLaurin, C.I.; Kress, M.A.; Kenney, J.A., Jr Incidence of common dermatoses in a predominantly black dermatologic practice. *Cutis,* **1983**, *32*(4), 388-390, 390.
[PMID: 6226496]

[41]   Taylor, S.C.; Cook-Bolden, F.; Rahman, Z.; Strachan, D. Acne vulgaris in skin of color. *J. Am. Acad. Dermatol.,* **2002**, *46*(2) Suppl Understanding, S98-S106.
[http://dx.doi.org/10.1067/mjd.2002.120791] [PMID: 11807471]

[42]   Passeron, T.; Nouveau, S.; Duval, C.; Cardot-Leccia, N.; Piffaut, V.; Bourreau, E.; Queille-Roussel, C.; Bernerd, F. Development and validation of a reproducible model for studying post-inflammatory hyperpigmentation. *Pigment Cell Melanoma Res.,* **2018**, *31*(5), 649-652.
[http://dx.doi.org/10.1111/pcmr.12692] [PMID: 29436173]

[43]   Sheth, V.M.; Pandya, A.G. Melasma: a comprehensive update: part I. *J. Am. Acad. Dermatol.,* **2011**, *65*(4), 689-697.
[http://dx.doi.org/10.1016/j.jaad.2010.12.046] [PMID: 21920241]

[44]   Khanna, N.; Rasool, S. Facial melanoses: Indian perspective. *Indian J. Dermatol. Venereol. Leprol.,* **2011**, *77*(5), 552-563.
[http://dx.doi.org/10.4103/0378-6323.84046] [PMID: 21860153]

[45]   Sarkar, R.; Jagadeesan, S.; Basavapura Madegowda, S.; Verma, S.; Hassan, I.; Bhat, Y.; Minni, K.; Jha, A.; Das, A.; Jain, G.; Arya, L.; Mandlewala, Z.; Bagadia, J.; Garg, V. Clinical and epidemiologic features of melasma: a multicentric cross-sectional study from India. *Int. J. Dermatol.,* **2019**, *58*(11), 1305-1310.
[http://dx.doi.org/10.1111/ijd.14541] [PMID: 31187480]

[46]   Rhodes, A.R.; Harrist, T.J.; Momtaz-T, K. The PUVA-induced pigmented macule: a lentiginous proliferation of large, sometimes cytologically atypical, melanocytes. *J. Am. Acad. Dermatol.,* **1983**, *9*(1), 47-58.
[http://dx.doi.org/10.1016/S0190-9622(83)70106-4] [PMID: 6411778]

[47]   Rhodes, A.R.; Albert, L.S.; Barnhill, R.L.; Weinstock, M.A. Sun-induced freckles in children and young adults. A correlation of clinical and histopathologic features. *Cancer,* **1991**, *67*(7), 1990-2001.
[http://dx.doi.org/10.1002/1097-0142(19910401)67:7<1990::AID-CNCR2820670728>3.0.CO;2-P]
[PMID: 2004316]

[48]   Bliss, J.M.; Ford, D.; Swerdlow, A.J.; Armstrong, B.K.; Cristofolini, M.; Elwood, J.M.; Green, A.; Holly, E.A.; Mack, T.; MacKie, R.M. The International Melanoma Analysis Group (IMAGE). Risk of cutaneous melanoma associated with pigmentation characteristics and freckling: systematic overview of 10 case-control studies. *Int. J. Cancer,* **1995**, *62*(4), 367-376.
[http://dx.doi.org/10.1002/ijc.2910620402] [PMID: 7635560]

[49]   Kanwar, A.J.; Dogra, S.; Handa, S.; Parsad, D.; Radotra, B.D. A study of 124 Indian patients with lichen planus pigmentosus. *Clin. Exp. Dermatol.,* **2003**, *28*(5), 481-485.
[http://dx.doi.org/10.1046/j.1365-2230.2003.01367.x] [PMID: 12950331]

[50]   Mulinari-Brenner, F.A.; Guilherme, M.R.; Peretti, M.C.; Werner, B. Frontal fibrosing alopecia and lichen planus pigmentosus: diagnosis and therapeutic challenge. *An. Bras. Dermatol.,* **2017**, *92*(5) Suppl. 1, 79-81.
[http://dx.doi.org/10.1590/abd1806-4841.20175833] [PMID: 29267454]

[51]   Bishnoi, A.; Parsad, D.; Saikia, U.N.; Kumaran, M.S. Coexistence of Linear and Inversus Variants of Lichen Planus Pigmentosus: A Rare Occurrence. *Indian J. Dermatol.,* **2019**, *64*(2), 152-154.
[http://dx.doi.org/10.4103/ijd.IJD_599_17] [PMID: 30983614]

[52]   Bahadir, S.; Cobanoglu, U.; Cimsit, G.; Yayli, S.; Alpay, K. Erythema dyschromicum perstans: response to dapsone therapy. *Int. J. Dermatol.,* **2004**, *43*(3), 220-222.
[http://dx.doi.org/10.1111/j.1365-4632.2004.01984.x] [PMID: 15009398]

[53]   Tienthavorn, T.; Tresukosol, P.; Sudtikoonaseth, P. Patch testing and histopathology in Thai patients with hyperpigmentation due to Erythema dyschromicum perstans, Lichen planus pigmentosus, and pigmented contact dermatitis. *Asian Pac. J. Allergy Immunol.,* **2014**, *32*(2), 185-192.
[PMID: 25003734]

[54]   Lin, S.H.; Ho, J.C.; Cheng, Y.W.; Huang, P.H.; Wang, C.Y. Prurigo pigmentosa: a clinical and histopathologic study of 11 cases. *Chang Gung Med. J.,* **2010**, *33*(2), 157-163.
[PMID: 20438668]

[55]   Chao, L.L.; Lu, C.F.; Shih, C.M. Molecular detection and genetic identification of Borrelia garinii and Borrelia afzelii from patients presenting with a rare skin manifestation of prurigo pigmentosa in Taiwan. *Int. J. Infect. Dis.,* **2013**, *17*(12), e1141-e1147.
[http://dx.doi.org/10.1016/j.ijid.2013.08.004] [PMID: 24103333]

[56]   Baumann, L.; Rodriguez, D.; Taylor, S.C.; Wu, J. Natural considerations for skin of color. *Cutis,* **2006**, *78*(6) Suppl., 2-19.
[PMID: 17354519]

[57]   Watanabe, S.; Nakai, K.; Ohnishi, T. Condition known as "dark rings under the eyes" in the Japanese population is a kind of dermal melanocytosis which can be successfully treated by Q-switched ruby laser. *Dermatol. Surg.,* **2006**, *32*(6), 785-789.
[PMID: 16792642]

[58]   Sinha, S.; Schwartz, R.A. Juvenile acanthosis nigricans. *J. Am. Acad. Dermatol.,* **2007**, *57*(3), 502-508.
[http://dx.doi.org/10.1016/j.jaad.2006.08.016] [PMID: 17592743]

[59]   Adigun, C.G.; Pandya, A.G. Improvement of idiopathic acanthosis nigricans with a triple combination depigmenting cream. *J. Eur. Acad. Dermatol. Venereol.,* **2009**, *23*(4), 486-487.
[http://dx.doi.org/10.1111/j.1468-3083.2008.02931.x] [PMID: 18721216]

[60]   Chan, H.H.; Leung, R.S.; Ying, S.Y. A retrospective analysis of complications in the treatment of nevus of Ota with the Q-switched alexandrite and Q-switched Nd:YAG lasers. *Dermatol Surg,* **2000**, *26*, 1000-6.

[61]   Chan, H.H.; Ying, S.Y.; Ho, W.S. An *in vivo* trial comparing the clinical efficacy and complications of Q-switched 755 nm alexandrite and Q-switched 1064 nm Nd:YAG lasers in the treatment of nevus of Ota. *Dermatol Surg,* **2000**, *26*, 919-22.

[62]   Levin, C.Y.; Maibach, H. Exogenous ochronosis. An update on clinical features, causative agents and treatment options. *Am. J. Clin. Dermatol.,* **2001**, *2*(4), 213-217.
[http://dx.doi.org/10.2165/00128071-200102040-00002] [PMID: 11705248]

[63]   Zawar, V.P.; Mhaskar, S.T. Exogenous ochronosis following hydroquinone for melasma. *J. Cosmet. Dermatol.,* **2004**, *3*(4), 234-236.
[http://dx.doi.org/10.1111/j.1473-2130.2004.00089.x] [PMID: 17166112]

[64]   Charlín, R.; Barcaui, C.B.; Kac, B.K.; Soares, D.B.; Rabello-Fonseca, R.; Azulay-Abulafia, L. Hydroquinone-induced exogenous ochronosis: a report of four cases and usefulness of dermoscopy. *Int. J. Dermatol.,* **2008**, *47*(1), 19-23.
[http://dx.doi.org/10.1111/j.1365-4632.2007.03351.x] [PMID: 18173595]

CHAPTER 5

Prevalence of Pigmentary Disorders and their Impact on the Quality of Life

Abstract: Melasma, vitiligo, lentigos, post inflammatory hyperpigmentation are the most common pigmentary disorders, which are caused by the altered production and distribution of melanin in the skin. Various intrinsic and extrinsic factors including ultraviolet radiation, food, chemical, certain medications, hormones *etc.* are responsible for affecting pigment cell functions with an altered amount of melanin pigment. As a result, pigmentation disorders are caused, which may be either hyperpigmentation or hypopigmentation. These are commonly seen in dermatology practice and can have a negative psychosocial impact on human life. In spite being of cosmetic concern, these disorders are devastating and stigmatizing; hence, there is an urgent need for effective treatment of pigmentary disorders based on their prevalence and impact on the quality of life. Prevalence of pigmentary disorders has been assessed in many countries of the world. In the present chapter, we have discussed about the prevalence of pigmentary disorders with their impact on quality of life and social status of an individual.

Keywords : Dermatology, Pigmentary disorders, Prevalence, Psychosocial, Quality of life.

1. INTRODUCTION

Vitiligo, melasma, idiopathic guttate hypomelanosis (IGH), lentigos and post inflammatory hyperpigmentation (PIH) are commonly occurring pigmentary disorders. These disorders are caused by the increase or decrease of melanin in the skin [1, 2]. Vitiligo, IGH appear as hypopigmented or lighter areas on the skin whereas melasma, PIH, lentigos appear as hyperpigmented or darker areas. Ultraviolet light and various hormones are responsible for affecting pigment cell function and proliferation and create altered pigmentation in the form of melasma and lentigo [3]. PIH is an excess of melanin in the skin, which is developed after an inflammatory dermatosis. It is caused when there is an increase in melanin synthesis in the epidermis during inflammation and can cover diffused areas based on the location of inflammation whereas in vitiligo, an autoimmune response is found [4].

Pigmentary disorders including PIH, lentigo, melasma, vitiligo, IGH are the leading five skin conditions seen by the dermatologists all over the world. Among the population of almost every country, there is an obsession of looking stunner, and this has greatly affected the social status of an individual [5]. Studies have shown that pigmentary disorders can affect an individual psychologically and emotionally, and also brutally affect the patient's health related quality of life. Hyper or hypo pigmented spots on the face are often psychologically devastating. They result in cosmetic disfigurement and influence psychosocial and psychosexual identity of the patient. Skin color stratification, differentiation by lightness or darkness of skin tone, continues to be a significant sociological issue in the world [6].

The prevalence of pigmentary disorders has been assessed in many countries of the world. True prevalence of pigmentary disorders in any particular area cannot be determined until large epidemiological studies have been done. Rate of prevalence may vary in different countries and depends on racial variations. Prevalence can be expressed by the data collected from the patients of pigmentary disorders in medical and dermatology clinics. Despite various treatment strategies including noncytotoxic laser, topical formulations, chemical peeling and skin grafting have been practised by the dermatologists and cosmetologists, the impact of pigmentary disorders remains dreadful [7 - 9].

There is limited literature available citing the prevalence of pigmentary disorders. Pigmentary disorders substantially create psychological and emotional burden on patients and rigorously affect the health related quality of life of the patient. In the present chapter, we have discussed the various studies conducted in different parts of the world to found out the prevalence of pigmentary disorders including hyperpigmentary disorders and hypopigmentary disorders. Additionally, we have discussed the impact of pigmentary disorders on the socioeconomic behaviour and quality of life of the patient suffering from these diseases.

2. STUDIES CONDUCTED TO DETERMINE THE PREVALENCE OF PIGMENTARY DISORDERS IN DIFFERENT COUNTRIES

Halder *et al.* [10] reported an incidence of common dermatoses including pigmentary disorders in African Americans and Caucasians. Pigmentary disorders were found more prevalent in dark skinned people than in white skinned people. Another similar study was conducted by Chua-Ty *et al.* [11] on Chinese, Indians, Malaysians and other population who lived in Singapore. Prevalence of pigmentary disorders was found to be 1.8% Chinese, 2.7% Malaysian, 2.3% Indian and 1.2% in others. Malaysian population was found to be more prevalent followed by Indian population in Singapore. A study conducted in Kuwait determined the spectrum and pattern of pigmentary disorders in children from Kuwait. Among the total 10,000 patients studied, 96% were Arab descents.

Psoriasis (4%), pityriasis alba (5.2%) and vitiligo were the common skin problems found in child patients [12]. Similarly, Gul *et al.* [13] have also studied the spectrum of dermatologic problems in child patients of Turkey and found that pigmentation disorders were prevalent in 3.8% patients among the patients studied [13]. But in another study conducted in Turkey , there were 17.2% child patients who suffered from pigmentation disorders among the total 1932 patients analysed [14]. Various other studies have also reported the epidemiology of pigmentary disorders in pediatric patients of different other countries [15 - 18].

Child *et al.* [19] have studied the spectrum of skin diseases occurred in dark skinned population in south-east London. Psoriasis and post inflammatory hyperpigmentation were the common pigmentary disorders found in black skin. Their study demonstrated the wide spectrum of skin diseases and disorders more common in black people. Pigmentary disorders were more prevalent in adult population than in children under study. Hartshorne [20] have conducted a survey based study of 7029 patients in Johannesburg area, South Africa. Among all the patients studied, 76% were black, 10% were white, 6.7% Indian and 6.1% were mixed race. Psoriasis (9.6%) was found in the Indian race and eczema, acne, warts are the common skin problems of black, white and mixed races.

Dunwell and Rose [21] have retrospectively studied the spectrum of skin diseases in one thousand patients of Afro-Carribean population in Kingston, Jamaica. Pigmentary disorders including psoriasis, melasma, solar lentigos and post inflammatory hyperpigmentation were seen in 16.56% patients. Acne and eczema were the most common skin problems found in this population. Another study on the same race was conducted in Paris region by Arsouze *et al.* [22]. Dermatological conditions of black patients of phototype V and VI were studied and about 25% cases were associated with dyschromia. Their study emphasized on the prevalence of skin diseases more specific to black population such as dyschromia and other pigmentary diseases.

A survey based study was conducted by El-Essawi *et al.* [23] in Arab Americans of Detroit, Michigan to estimate the pattern of skin diseases. The most common skin conditions were acne, eczema, warts and melasma. Melasma is among the other pigmentary disorder more commonly found in that population. They have concluded that the skin related issues that affect Arab Americans were similar to those which affect other skin of color. Likewise, Taylor *et al.* [24] have conducted a cohort study on 140 patients undergoing skin exams at a private dermatology clinic in North Carolina. Around 80% of the patients were diagnosed with pigmentary disorders. Most of the patients with pigmentary disorders had solar lentigos (74.3%) followed by IGH (10.7%), post inflammatory hyperpigmentation (5.7%), melasma (3.5%), vitiligo (0.7%). About 15% of the patients were not only having single pigmentation disorders rather they had multiple pigmentation problems.

An interesting study conducted by Werlinger *et al.* [25] assessed the prevalence of self diagnosed melasma among premenopausal Latino women in Dallas and Fort Worth, Texas. The women subjects were interviewed by telephone. The prevalence rate of melasma was 8.8%, which included subjects who told that they had melasma at the time of telephonic interview. An additional 4% subjects had melasma in the past. Their study concluded that Dallas residents had four times more risk of melasma than people of Fort Worth. To assess the prevalence of melasma in Chinese Han and Chinese Yi community of Liangshan district, China, an analogous community based study was conducted by Wang *et al.* [26]. The prevalence of melasma in Chinese Yi (21.43%) was found significantly higher than Chinese Han (9.7%). Significantly higher prevalence of melasma was found in Chinese Yi males and females than Chinese Han males and females. The prevalence rate was higher in females than in males of both the community.

A study conducted by Ranu *et al.* [27] has assessed the prevalence of periorbital hyperpigmentation (POH) in Singapore. One thousand consecutive patients were assessed for POH, among them 200 patients were investigated to define causes of POH. Patients include Chinese, Malaysians and Indians. The most common form of POH noted was vascular type (41.8%) followed by constitutional (38.6%) and post inflammatory hyperpigmentation (12%).The vascular type was prevalent in Chinese and constitutional was predominant in Indians and Malaysians.

Sheth *et al.* [28] have published their study on the prevalence of periorbital hyperpigmentation (POH) in Gujarat region of India. Two hundred patients were included in the study, all were subjected to careful Wood's lamp examination, eyelid stretch and laboratory investigation. Periorbital hyperpigmentation was most prevalent in 16-25 years aged patients (47.5%), in females (81%). Common form of POH is constitutional (51.50%) followed by Post inflammatory hyperpigmentation (22.50%). Wood's lamp examination revealed POH to be dermal in 60.5%. Grade 2 POH was found in 58% patients. Faulty habits such as lack of proper sleep (40%), frequent use of cosmetics (36.5%), and frequent eye rubbing (32.5%) were noted. Association of POH with stress (71%), family history (63%) and atrophy (33%) was observed.

In India, vitiligo has been considered as social stigma. In order to assess the profile of vitiligo, Agrawal *et al.* [29] have presented a profile of vitiligo in Kumaun region of Uttarakhand, India. 762 vitiligo patients from outpatient department of dermatology of Government Medical College, Haldwani, Kumaun, Uttarakhand were examined for the onset of disease, form of vitiligo, site of onset *etc*. They have concluded that the onset of vitiligo was most common in patients aged 0-10 years. The most common type of vitiligo was acrofacial type, followed by vitiligo vulgaris, focal, segmental mucosal, and universal vitiligo. Common site of onset was lower limbs followed by head, neck, upper limbs, trunk, genitalia and mucasae.

In order to assess the world prevalence of vitiligo, Zhang *et al*. [30] have conducted a meta analysis in which total 103 studies containing 82 population based studies and 22 hospital based studies were included. Countries where the prevalence of vitiligo has been assessed in the studies were India, Denmark, Sri Lanka, China, Sweden, USA, Fareo Island, Tanzania, France, Egypt, Turkey, Nepal, Iran, Korea, Mexico, Kuwait, Nigeria, Japan, Jordan, Saudi Arabia, Germany, Italy and the areas covered Africa, Asia, America, Oceania, Europe and Atlantic. Vitiligo prevalence ranged from 0.004% to 9.98%. The prevalence of vitiligo in different areas was 0.1% in Asia, 0.2% in America, 0.1% in Atlantic, and 0.4% in Africa. They have concluded that the high prevalence of vitiligo was found in Africa and in females.

Recently Rendon [31] has described the status of hyperpigmentation in patients of Hispanic population, which is the third largest growing population in United States. Hispanics were found to be more susceptible to a variety of pigmentation disorders including post inflammatory hyperpigmentation and melasma. He has used various treatment strategies including microdermabrasion, chemical peeling, laser, use of skin lightening agents to treat hyperpigmentation.

3. IMPACT OF PIGMENTARY DISORDERS ON QUALITY OF LIFE OF THE PATIENT

In a human population of almost all countries of the world, there is an obsession of looking their skin healthy, bright and spotless. This greatly affects the social standing of an individual. Studies have shown that disturbance in the skin texture in the form of pigmentary disorders can affect a person psychologically and emotionally and also affect the patient's quality of life. There were various studies which showed that the patients with vitiligo and other pigmentary disorders were concerned with stigmatism, depression, and its affects the health related quality of life [32 - 50].

Bae *et al*. [51] have conducted questionnaire based study to assessed factors affecting quality of life in patients with vitiligo. Total 1123 vitiligo patients were studied in which 609 were male and 514 were females, recruited from 21 hospitals in Korea. Data were collected by using structured questionnaire and the Skindex-29 instrument. Their results showed that quality of life of patients aged

20-59 years, who have more active life than older patients, was associated with functional impairment. The patients with higher educational background were associated with emotional impairment. Similarly an institutional based case control study was conducted to evaluate the psychiatric mobility in 61 patients of vitiligo and to assess the morbidity in eight dimensions including fear, discomfort, cognitive, social, depression, limitation, anger and embarrassment. Self reporting questionnaire and Skindex were used to assess the results which showed that maximum association with psychiatric morbidity was seen in acral vitiligo (86.67%) followed by vitiligo vulgaris (68%) and mucosal vitiligo (62.5%). Depression (62.29%) was the most common psychiatric morbidity in vitiligo patients followed by embarrassment (55.73%), social problem (54.09%), cognitive impairment (50.81%), physical limitation (47.54%), discomfort (40.98%), anger (36.06%) and fear (24.59%) [52].

In order to establish the prevalence of psychological comorbidity in vitiligo patients, Osinubi *et al.* [53] have performed a comprehensive literature search and identified 29 studies with 2530 patients of vitiligo. From this, they have found that a range of psychological outcomes were common in vitiligo cases. The prevalence of anxiety and depression was found influenced by the type of screening tools used by the researchers in their studies. When specific tools were used, the prevalence of clinically diagnosed depression and anxiety was low. But, when non specific tools were used, the prevalence remained similar for depression and increased for anxiety.

The meta analysis review by Wang *et al.* [54] also showed the prevalence and odd of depression in patients of vitiligo. 1965 patients were identified from 20 cohort studies. The prevalence of depression was 29% across 17 populations. Vitiligo patients were 4.96 times more likely to display depression compared with controls. Significantly, the prevalence of depression in Asian and female patients with vitiligo was higher than in Caucasian and male. With Hamilton Depression Rating Scale (HDRS) questionnaire, the pooled prevalence of depressive symptoms was higher and the heterogeneity was lowered, in comparison with other questionnaires.

Sawant *et al.* [55] have recently studied gender difference in depression, coping, stigma and quality of life in vitiligo patients. A total of 156 patients were screened. They have collected the desired information with the administration of participation scale, Beck's depression inventory, dermatology life quality index, chronic skin disease questionnaire. The prevalence of depression was 63.64% in females and 42.86% in males. On participation scale, no significant differences were seen though 52% females have stigmatized as compared to 45% males. Whereas almost 97% of the patients had impaired quality of life and there was no significant difference in both gender on total score. There was significantly higher coping style in females than in males with significant difference in total score.

Besides psychiatric morbidity in patients of vitiligo, there was a prevalence of psychological issues with patients of melasma also, which affects the quality of life of the patients. Yalamanchili *et al*. [56] have conducted a clinico-epidemiological study and quality of life assessment. Quality of life was assessed by MELASQOL scale with standard structured questionnaire. Total 140 cases were studied in which 69.7% were females and 32% were males. The mean MELASQOL score was calculated as 28.8, with most patients reporting frustration and embarrassment. Two different cross sectional studies were done with 85 women and 49 women diagnosed with melasma in southern Brazil and Singapore respectively. Quality of life assessment was done using melasma quality of life scale and dermatology life quality index questionnaires. Both the studies contribute in evaluating the effect of melasma on quality of life of the women patients of Southern Brazil and Singapore [57, 58].

Pollo *et al* [59] have enrolled 155 adults with melasma for their study to assessed the factors such as sex, marital status, education and income associated with quality of life of the patients. Influence of these factors on MelasQol score was studied. In melasma patients, the perception of quality of life impairment was influenced by low family income, low scholarly, single marital status and greater clinical severity. Similarly, Deshpande *et al*. [60] have also conducted a cross sectional study of psychiatric morbidity in patients of melasma. Their study involved 55 patients of melasma. Cases of melasma were assessed by International classification of diseases-10 diagnostic criteria for research, hospital anxiety depression scale *etc*. The most common psychiatric morbidity found in their study was depressive disorder.

Dabas *et al*. [61] have conducted a cross sectional study to assessed the psychological disturbance in patients of pigmentary disorders. Their study involved 100 patients of melasma, acquired dermal macular hyperpigmentation (ADMH) and vitiligo. PRIME-MD patient health questionnaire, dermatology life quality index, generalized anxiety disorders-7, patient health questionnaire- 9 and patient health questionnaire-15 were used for the estimation of quality of life, depression, psychiatric comorbidities, general anxiety and somatoform disorders and correlated with age, gender, marital status, occupation, severity and progression of pigmentary diseases. The patients with melasma, vitiligo, and ADMH have shown the prevalence of anxiety disorder as 11.6%, 21% and 18% respectively. Depression was more common in vitiligo (27%) as compared to ADMH (24.1%) and melasma (12.85). Somatoform disorder was seen in 17.9%, 14.3%, 8.1% patients with vitiligo, ADMH and melasma respectively.

CONCLUSION

Pigmentary disorders are prevalent in many countries of the world and also pose emotional and psychological burden on patients and severely affect patients health related quality of life. Vitiligo, post inflammatory hyperpigmentation, melasma, lentigines *etc.* are the various pigmentary disorders which appear as social stigma rather than diseases. Although, these diseases pose a significant negative impact on the quality of life of the patient, still patients do not receive sufficient treatment for their disease. Thus, there is a need for effective treatments based on the prevalence and effects of pigmentary disorders. When prescribing any medications, the healthcare providers should consider the impact of pigmentary disorders on health related quality of life of the patients. Additionally, there is a need to counsel patients about their disease condition and its possible treatments, through psychological and confidence boosting sessions.

REFERENCES

[1]   Sugumaran, M. Comparative biochemistry of eumelanogenesis and the protective roles of phenoloxidase and melanin in insects. *Pigment Cell Res.,* **2002**, *15*(1), 2-9.
[http://dx.doi.org/10.1034/j.1600-0749.2002.00056.x] [PMID: 11837452]

[2]   Li, Y.; Huang, J.; Lu, J.; Ding, Y.; Jiang, L.; Hu, S.; Chen, J.; Zeng, Q. The role and mechanism of Asian medicinal plants in treating skin pigmentary disorders. *J. Ethnopharmacol.,* **2019**, *245*, 112173.
[http://dx.doi.org/10.1016/j.jep.2019.112173] [PMID: 31445129]

[3]   Svobodová, A.; Vostálová, J. Solar radiation induced skin damage: review of protective and preventive options. *Int. J. Radiat. Biol.,* **2010**, *86*(12), 999-1030.
[http://dx.doi.org/10.3109/09553002.2010.501842] [PMID: 20807180]

[4]   Siebenga, P.S.; van Amerongen, G.; Klaassen, E.S.; de Kam, M.L.; Rissmann, R.; Groeneveld, G.J. The ultraviolet B inflammation model: Postinflammatory hyperpigmentation and validation of a reduced UVB exposure paradigm for inducing hyperalgesia in healthy subjects. *Eur. J. Pain,* **2019**, *23*(5), 874-883.
[http://dx.doi.org/10.1002/ejp.1353] [PMID: 30597682]

[5]   Picardi, A.; Abeni, D.; Renzi, C.; Braga, M.; Melchi, C.F.; Pasquini, P. Treatment outcome and incidence of psychiatric disorders in dermatological out-patients. *J. Eur. Acad. Dermatol. Venereol.,* **2003**, *17*(2), 155-159.
[http://dx.doi.org/10.1046/j.1468-3083.2003.00619.x] [PMID: 12705743]

[6]   Hourblin, V.; Nouveau, S.; Roy, N.; de Lacharrière, O. Skin complexion and pigmentary disorders in facial skin of 1204 women in 4 Indian cities. *Indian J. Dermatol. Venereol. Leprol.,* **2014**, *80*(5), 395-401.
[http://dx.doi.org/10.4103/0378-6323.140290] [PMID: 25201838]

[7]   Del Giudice, P.; Raynaud, E.; Mahé, A. [Cosmetic use of skin depigmentation products in Africa]. *Bull. Soc. Pathol. Exot.,* **2003**, *96*(5), 389-393.
[PMID: 15015845]

[8]   Pasricha, J.S.; Khaitan, B.K.; Dash, S. Pigmentary disorders in India. *Dermatol. Clin.,* **2007**, *25*(3), 343-352, viii.
[http://dx.doi.org/10.1016/j.det.2007.05.004] [PMID: 17662900]

[9]   Armenta, A.M.; Henkel, E.D.; Ahmed, A.M. Pigmentation disorders in the elderly. *Drugs Aging,*

2019, *36*(3), 235-245.
[http://dx.doi.org/10.1007/s40266-018-00633-w] [PMID: 30637685]

[10]   Halder, R.M.; Grimes, P.E.; McLaurin, C.I.; Kress, M.A.; Kenney, J.A., Jr Incidence of common dermatoses in a predominantly black dermatologic practice. *Cutis,* **1983**, *32*(4), 388-390, 390.
[PMID: 6226496]

[11]   Chua-Ty, G.; Goh, C.L.; Koh, S.L. Pattern of skin diseases at the national skin centre (Singapore) from 1989–1990. *Int. J. Dermatol.,* **1992**, *31*(8), 555-559.
[http://dx.doi.org/10.1111/j.1365-4362.1992.tb02717.x] [PMID: 1428445]

[12]   Nanda, A.; Al-Hasawi, F.; Alsaleh, Q.A. A prospective survey of pediatric dermatology clinic patients in Kuwait: an analysis of 10,000 cases. *Pediatr. Dermatol.,* **1999**, *16*(1), 6-11.
[http://dx.doi.org/10.1046/j.1525-1470.1999.99002.x] [PMID: 10027990]

[13]   Gül, U.; Cakmak, S.K.; Gönül, M.; Kiliç, A.; Bilgili, S. Pediatric skin disorders encountered in a dermatology outpatient clinic in Turkey. *Pediatr. Dermatol.,* **2008**, *25*(2), 277-278.
[http://dx.doi.org/10.1111/j.1525-1470.2008.00656.x] [PMID: 18429805]

[14]   Sula, B.; Uçmak, D.; Saka, G.; Akdeniz, S.; Yavuz, E.; Yakut, Y.; Arslan, E.; Aktaş, H.; Yıldız, M.; Yolbir, S.; Azizoğlu, R. Prevalence of skin disorders among primary school children in Diyarbakir, Turkey. *Arch. Argent. Pediatr.,* **2014**, *112*(5), 434-438.
[PMID: 25192524]

[15]   Ogunbiyi, A.O.; Owoaje, E.; Ndahi, A. Prevalence of skin disorders in school children in Ibadan, Nigeria. *Pediatr. Dermatol.,* **2005**, *22*(1), 6-10.
[http://dx.doi.org/10.1111/j.1525-1470.2005.22101.x] [PMID: 15660888]

[16]   Ogunbiyi, A.O.; Omigbodun, Y.; Owoaje, E. Prevalence of skin disorders in school children in southwest Nigeria. *Int. J. Adolesc. Med. Health,* **2009**, *21*(2), 235-241.
[http://dx.doi.org/10.1515/IJAMH.2009.21.2.235] [PMID: 19702203]

[17]   Komba, E.V.; Mgonda, Y.M. The spectrum of dermatological disorders among primary school children in Dar es Salaam. *BMC Public Health,* **2010**, *10*, 765.
[http://dx.doi.org/10.1186/1471-2458-10-765] [PMID: 21162714]

[18]   Amin, T.T.; Ali, A.; Kaliyadan, F. Skin disorders among male primary school children in Al Hassa, Saudi Arabia: prevalence and socio-demographic correlates--a comparison of urban and rural populations. *Rural Remote Health,* **2011**, *11*(1), 1517.
[PMID: 21355670]

[19]   Child, F.J.; Fuller, L.C.; Higgins, E.M.; Du Vivier, A.W. A study of the spectrum of skin disease occurring in a black population in south-east London. *Br. J. Dermatol.,* **1999**, *141*(3), 512-517.
[http://dx.doi.org/10.1046/j.1365-2133.1999.03047.x] [PMID: 10583057]

[20]   Hartshorne, S.T. Dermatological disorders in Johannesburg, South Africa. *Clin. Exp. Dermatol.,* **2003**, *28*(6), 661-665.
[http://dx.doi.org/10.1046/j.1365-2230.2003.01417.x] [PMID: 14616837]

[21]   Dunwell, P.; Rose, A. Study of the skin disease spectrum occurring in an Afro-Caribbean population. *Int. J. Dermatol.,* **2003**, *42*(4), 287-289.
[http://dx.doi.org/10.1046/j.1365-4362.2003.01358.x] [PMID: 12694494]

[22]   Arsouze, A.; Fitoussi, C.; Cabotin, P.P.; Chaine, B.; Delebecque, C.; Raynaud, E.; Kornfeld, S.; Dehen, L.; Bafounta, M.L.; Bourgeois-Droin, C.; Dubertret, L.; Dupuy, A.; Petit, A. [Presenting skin disorders in black Afro-Caribbean patients: a multicentre study conducted in the Paris region]. *Ann. Dermatol. Venereol.,* **2008**, *135*(3), 177-182.
[http://dx.doi.org/10.1016/j.annder.2007.11.008] [PMID: 18374847]

[23]   El-Essawi, D.; Musial, J.L.; Hammad, A.; Lim, H.W. A survey of skin disease and skin-related issues in Arab Americans. *J. Am. Acad. Dermatol.,* **2007**, *56*(6), 933-938.
[http://dx.doi.org/10.1016/j.jaad.2007.01.031] [PMID: 17321004]

[24]   Taylor, A.; Pawaskar, M.; Taylor, S.L.; Balkrishnan, R.; Feldman, S.R. Prevalence of pigmentary disorders and their impact on quality of life: a prospective cohort study. *J. Cosmet. Dermatol.,* **2008**, *7*(3), 164-168.
[http://dx.doi.org/10.1111/j.1473-2165.2008.00384.x] [PMID: 18789050]

[25]   Werlinger, K.D.; Guevara, I.L.; González, C.M.; Rincón, E.T.; Caetano, R.; Haley, R.W.; Pandya, A.G. Prevalence of self-diagnosed melasma among premenopausal Latino women in Dallas and Fort Worth, Tex. *Arch. Dermatol.,* **2007**, *143*(3), 424-425.
[http://dx.doi.org/10.1001/archderm.143.3.424] [PMID: 17372115]

[26]   Wang, R.L.; Wang, T.L.; Cao, L.S.; Shen, Y.W.; Cheng, Z.; Xiaolan, D.; DeQin, Z.; Bing, G. XingCai, Z.; Zhong, X.; Ying, T.; Zhong, Z.J. Prevalence of melasma in Chinese Han and Chinese Yi: a survey in Liangshan district. *Zhongguo Pifu Xingbingxue Zazhi,* **2010**, *24*(6), 546-548.

[27]   Ranu, H.; Thng, S.; Goh, B.K.; Burger, A.; Goh, C.L. Periorbital hyperpigmentation in Asians: an epidemiologic study and a proposed classification. *Dermatol. Surg.,* **2011**, *37*(9), 1297-1303.
[http://dx.doi.org/10.1111/j.1524-4725.2011.02065.x] [PMID: 21682796]

[28]   Sheth, P.B.; Shah, H.A.; Dave, J.N. Periorbital hyperpigmentation: a study of its prevalence, common causative factors and its association with personal habits and other disorders. *Indian J. Dermatol.,* **2014**, *59*(2), 151-157.
[http://dx.doi.org/10.4103/0019-5154.127675] [PMID: 24700933]

[29]   Agarwal, S.; Ojha, A.; Gupta, S. Profile of vitiligo in kumaun region of uttarakhand, India. *Indian J. Dermatol.,* **2014**, *59*(2), 209.
[http://dx.doi.org/10.4103/0019-5154.127706] [PMID: 24700953]

[30]   Zhang, Y.; Cai, Y.; Shi, M.; Jiang, S.; Cui, S.; Wu, Y.; Gao, X.H.; Chen, H.D. The Prevalence of Vitiligo: A Meta-Analysis. *PLoS One,* **2016**, *11*(9), e0163806.
[http://dx.doi.org/10.1371/journal.pone.0163806] [PMID: 27673680]

[31]   Rendon, M.I. Hyperpigmentation Disorders in Hispanic Population in the United States. *J. Drugs Dermatol.,* **2019**, *18*(3), 112-114.

[32]   Kent, G. Correlates of perceived stigma in vitiligo. *Psychol. Health,* **1999**, *14*(2), 241-251.
[http://dx.doi.org/10.1080/08870449908407325]

[33]   Gieler, U.; Brosig, B.; Schneideretal, U. Vitiligo-coping behaviour. *Dermatol Psychosomatics,* **2000**, *1*(1), 6-10.

[34]   Picardi, A.; Abeni, D.; Renzi, C.; Braga, M.; Puddu, P.; Pasquini, P. Increased psychiatric morbidity in female outpatients with skin lesions on visible parts of the body. *Acta Derm. Venereol.,* **2001**, *81*(6), 410-414.
[http://dx.doi.org/10.1046/j.1468-3083.2001.00336.x] [PMID: 11859943]

[35]   Mattoo, S.K.; Handa, S.; Kaur, I.; Gupta, N.; Malhotra, R. Psychiatric morbidity in vitiligo: prevalence and correlates in India. *J. Eur. Acad. Dermatol. Venereol.,* **2002**, *16*(6), 573-578.
[http://dx.doi.org/10.1046/j.1468-3083.2002.00590.x] [PMID: 12482039]

[36]   Parsad, D.; Pandhi, R.; Dogra, S.; Kanwar, A.J.; Kumar, B. Dermatology Life Quality Index score in vitiligo and its impact on the treatment outcome. *Br. J. Dermatol.,* **2003**, *148*(2), 373-374.
[http://dx.doi.org/10.1046/j.1365-2133.2003.05097_9.x] [PMID: 12588405]

[37]   Picardi, A.; Pasquini, P.; Cattaruzza, M.S.; Gaetano, P.; Melchi, C.F.; Baliva, G.; Camaioni, D.; Tiago, A.; Abeni, D.; Biondi, M. Stressful life events, social support, attachment security and alexithymia in vitiligo. A case-control study. *Psychother. Psychosom.,* **2003**, *72*(3), 150-158.
[http://dx.doi.org/10.1159/000069731] [PMID: 12707482]

[38]   Ongenae, K.; Van Geel, N.; De Schepper, S.; Naeyaert, J.M. Effect of vitiligo on self-reported health-related quality of life. *Br. J. Dermatol.,* **2005**, *152*(6), 1165-1172.
[http://dx.doi.org/10.1111/j.1365-2133.2005.06456.x] [PMID: 15948977]

[39]   Kim, D.Y.; Lee, J.W.; Whang, S.H.; Park, Y.K.; Hann, S.K.; Shin, Y.J. Quality of life for Korean patients with vitiligo: Skindex-29 and its correlation with clinical profiles. *J. Dermatol.,* **2009**, *36*(6), 317-322.
[http://dx.doi.org/10.1111/j.1346-8138.2009.00646.x] [PMID: 19500179]

[40]   Thompson, A.R.; Clarke, S.A.; Newell, R.J.; Gawkrodger, D.J. Appearance Research Collaboration (ARC). Vitiligo linked to stigmatization in British South Asian women: a qualitative study of the experiences of living with vitiligo. *Br. J. Dermatol.,* **2010**, *163*(3), 481-486.
[http://dx.doi.org/10.1111/j.1365-2133.2010.09828.x] [PMID: 20426784]

[41]   Bianchin, M.; Angrilli, A. Gender differences in emotional responses: a psychophysiological study. *Physiol. Behav.,* **2012**, *105*(4), 925-932.
[http://dx.doi.org/10.1016/j.physbeh.2011.10.031] [PMID: 22108508]

[42]   Pichaimuthu, R.; Ramaswamy, P.; Bikash, K.; Joseph, R. A measurement of the stigma among vitiligo and psoriasis patients in India. *Indian J. Dermatol. Venereol. Leprol.,* **2011**, *77*(3), 300-306.
[http://dx.doi.org/10.4103/0378-6323.79699] [PMID: 21508568]

[43]   Balaban, O.D.; Atagun, M.I.; Ozguven, H.D.; Ozsan, H.H. Psychiatric morbidity in patients with vitiligo. *Dusunen Adam: J Psy Neurol Sci,* **2011**, *6*, 306-313.
[http://dx.doi.org/10.5350/DAJPN2011240406]

[44]   Mishra, N.; Rastogi, M.K.; Gahalaut, P.; Agrawal, S. Dermatology specific quality of life in vitiligo patients and its relation with various variables: A hospital based cross sectional study. *J. Clin. Diagn. Res.,* **2014**, *8*(6), YC01-YC03.
[http://dx.doi.org/10.7860/JCDR/2014/8248.4508] [PMID: 25121050]

[45]   Sangma, L.N.; Nath, J.; Bhagabati, D. Quality of life and psychological morbidity in vitiligo patients: A study in a teaching hospital from north-east India. *Indian J Dermatol,* **2015**, *60*(2), 142-146.

[46]   Krüger, C.; Schallreuter, K.U. Stigmatisation, avoidance behaviour and difficulties in coping are common among adult patients with vitiligo. *Acta Derm. Venereol.,* **2015**, *95*(5), 553-558.
[http://dx.doi.org/10.2340/00015555-1981] [PMID: 25269389]

[47]   Deng, Y.; Chang, L.; Yang, M.; Huo, M.; Zhou, R.; Eder, A.B. Gender differences in emotional response: inconsistency between experience and expressivity. *PLoS One,* **2016**, *11*(6), e0158666.
[http://dx.doi.org/10.1371/journal.pone.0158666] [PMID: 27362361]

[48]   Lai, Y.C.; Yew, Y.W.; Kennedy, C.; Schwartz, R.A. Vitiligo and depression: a systematic review and meta-analysis of observational studies. *Br. J. Dermatol.,* **2017**, *177*(3), 708-718.
[http://dx.doi.org/10.1111/bjd.15199] [PMID: 27878819]

[49]   Sharma, V.K.; Bhatia, R. Vitiligo and the psyche. *Br. J. Dermatol.,* **2017**, *177*(3), 612-613.
[http://dx.doi.org/10.1111/bjd.15732] [PMID: 28940279]

[50]   Vernwal, D. A study of anxiety and depression in Vitiligo patients: New challenges to treat. *Eur. Psychiatry,* **2017**, *41*, S321.
[http://dx.doi.org/10.1016/j.eurpsy.2017.02.242]

[51]   Bae, J.M.; Lee, S.C.; Kim, T.H.; Yeom, S.D.; Shin, J.H.; Lee, W.J.; Lee, M.H.; Lee, A.Y.; Kim, K.H.; Kim, M.B.; Park, C.J.; Lee, S.H.; Kim, D.H.; Lee, H.J.; Lee, D.Y.; Choi, C.W.; Kim, Y.C.; Kang, H.Y.; Haw, S.; Lee, Y.B.; Yun, S.J.; Yun, S.K.; Hong, S.P.; Lee, Y.; Kim, H.J.; Choi, G.S. Factors affecting quality of life in patients with vitiligo: a nationwide study. *Br. J. Dermatol.,* **2018**, *178*(1), 238-244.
[http://dx.doi.org/10.1111/bjd.15560] [PMID: 28391642]

[52]   Sarkar, S.; Sarkar, T.; Sarkar, A.; Das, S. Vitiligo and psychiatric morbidity: A profile from a vitiligo clinic of a rural based tertiary care center of eastern India. *Indian J. Dermatol.,* **2018**, *63*(4), 281-284.
[http://dx.doi.org/10.4103/ijd.IJD_142_18] [PMID: 30078869]

[53]   Osinubi, O.; Grainge, M.J.; Hong, L.; Ahmed, A.; Batchelor, J.M.; Grindlay, D.; Thompson, A.R.; Ratib, S. The prevalence of psychological comorbidity in people with vitiligo: a systematic review and

meta-analysis. *Br. J. Dermatol.,* **2018,** *178*(4), 863-878.
[http://dx.doi.org/10.1111/bjd.16049] [PMID: 28991357]

[54] Wang, G.; Qiu, D.; Yang, H.; Liu, W. The prevalence and odds of depression in patients with vitiligo: a meta-analysis. *J. Eur. Acad. Dermatol. Venereol.,* **2018,** *32*(8), 1343-1351.
[http://dx.doi.org/10.1111/jdv.14739] [PMID: 29222958]

[55] Sawant, N.S.; Vanjari, N.A.; Khopkar, U. Gender differences in depression, coping, stigma, and quality of life in patients of vitiligo. *Dermatol. Res. Pract.,* **2019,** *2019*, 6879412.
[http://dx.doi.org/10.1155/2019/6879412] [PMID: 31065260]

[56] Yalamanchili, R.; Shastry, V.; Betkerur, J. Clinico-epidemiological Study and Quality of Life Assessment in Melasma. *Indian J. Dermatol.,* **2015,** *60*(5), 519.
[http://dx.doi.org/10.4103/0019-5154.164415] [PMID: 26538717]

[57] Freitag, F.M.; Cestari, T.F.; Leopoldo, L.R.; Paludo, P.; Boza, J.C. Effect of melasma on quality of life in a sample of women living in southern Brazil. *J. Eur. Acad. Dermatol. Venereol.,* **2008,** *22*(6), 655-662.
[http://dx.doi.org/10.1111/j.1468-3083.2007.02472.x] [PMID: 18410339]

[58] Harumi, O.; Goh, C.L. The Effect of Melasma on the Quality of Life in a Sample of Women Living in Singapore. *J. Clin. Aesthet. Dermatol.,* **2016,** *9*(1), 21-24.
[PMID: 26962388]

[59] Pollo, C.F.; Miot, L.D.B.; Meneguin, S.; Miot, H.A. Factors associated with quality of life in facial melasma: a cross-sectional study. *Int. J. Cosmet. Sci.,* **2018,** *40*(3), 313-316.
[http://dx.doi.org/10.1111/ics.12464] [PMID: 29734511]

[60] Deshpande, S.S.; Khatu, S.S.; Pardeshi, G.S.; Gokhale, N.R. Cross-sectional study of psychiatric morbidity in patients with melasma. *Indian J. Psychiatry,* **2018,** *60*(3), 324-328.
[http://dx.doi.org/10.4103/psychiatry.IndianJPsychiatry_115_16] [PMID: 30405259]

[61] Dabas, G.; Vinay, K.; Parsad, D.; Kumar, A.; Kumaran, M.S. Psychological disturbances in patients with pigmentary disorders: a cross-sectional study. *J. Eur. Acad. Dermatol. Venereol.,* **2019,** *34*(2), 392-399.
[http://dx.doi.org/10.1111/jdv.15987] [PMID: 31566833]

CHAPTER 6

Treatment and Therapies Available For Pigmentary Disorders

Abstract: Melanin is responsible for imparting color to the skin, hairs, eyes, and protecting the skin from harmful UV radiation. It is produced inside the specialized cells called melanocytes through a series of chemical and enzymatic reactions. However, due to the dysregulation of the factors responsible for melanin production, the irregular production and distribution of melanin occur, which lead to the onset of pigmentary disorders, such as hyperpigmentation or hypopigmentation. Pigmentary disorders are not always physically debilitating but have been associated with elevated psychosocial problems such as depression, frustration and anger. These psychosocial burdens in turn influence the quality of life and self-esteem. So, the treatment of pigmentation diseases appears as a growing concern to dermatologists today. Several treatment strategies including chemical peeling, stem cell transplant, topical treatment, laser therapy *etc.* have been unleashed in order to get rid of the problem. Hence, in the present chapter, we have discussed about the existing treatment options for pigmentation diseases practised by dermatologists all over the world.

Keywords : Dermatologists, Laser therapy, Melanin, Pigmentary disorders, Topical treatment.

1. INTRODUCTION

Melanin is the natural pigment responsible for imparting color to the skin, eyes and hairs as well as provides photoprotection of the skin against harmful UV radiation [1]. Melanogenesis is the process of production of melanin inside the specialized organelle called melanosomes of melanocytes, through a series of chemical and enzymatic reactions [2]. Irregular production and distribution of melanin into the skin leads to pigmentary disorders, which may be either hyperpigmentary disorders or hypopigmentary disorders. Hypo or hyper-pigmented lesions on the face or body causes a psychosocial problem in the patient and affect his social life. Public perception of healthy and attractive skin merged with the growing demand for treatment of pigmentation diseases provokes enormous interest pharmaceutically and cosmeceutically [3].

Although melanin is responsible for protecting skin from UV radiation but the production of surplus melanin and its distribution results in various hyperpig-

Sharique A. Ali & Naima Parveen

mentary diseases like melasma, post-inflammatory hyperpigmentation, solar lentigos, *etc*. Hyperpigmented macules or lesions of variable sizes are seen on the exposed areas of the body of the person suffering from hyperpigmentation diseases [4, 5]. Hypopigmentation is a general term used for any form of decreased or absent skin pigmentation. It may be acquired or congenital, localized or generalized and may occur as separated or be associated with a broad range of congenital or acquired disorders. Pigmentation of the skin normally differs according to the racial origin and the amount of sun exposure. Pigmentation disorders include the entities that are characterized by a pathological change in melanocytes [6].

Treatments available for hyperpigmentation include removal of stimulating factors, photoprotection, and pigment reduction with the topical formulation and/or physical approaches such as laser therapy, chemical peel, camouflage, dermabrasion [7]. Treatment for hypopigmentary diseases is diverse and depends on the cause of the disease. It involves topical application of corticosteroids; physical treatment involves light or laser therapy, surgical skin grafting *etc*. PUVA (psoralen and ultraviolet light) is the most commonly used treatment for hypopigmentation and is recommended as the first-line therapeutic strategy. Topical prescription medications are given for chronic hypopigmentation. Camouflaging with cosmetic tattooing or permanent makeup may be the best option for the form of hypopigmentation that is unresponsive to medications. But, overall depigmentation is the only option for the patient who experiences extreme hypopigmentation over half of their body [3, 7].

With increased psychosocial problems associated with the patients having pigmentation disorders, researchers are going on how to treat those diseases and what can make the skin looks stunning. As a result, many treatment options have been developed. So in the present chapter, we have discussed in detail the conventional and current treatment available for hypopigmentation and hyperpigmentation with their variable efficacies.

2. TREATMENTS AVAILABLE FOR HYPOPIGMENTATION

The main objective of the treatment is to control the degeneration of melanocytes and stimulates its migration and distribution to surrounding cells. Conventional treatment for hypopigmentation such as topical treatment and physical or photo-therapy remains the basis of modern treatment. Treatment strategies are broadly categorized into physical, pharmacological and surgical.

2.1. Physical Treatment

Physical treatment includes utilization of light or radiation such as ultraviolet radiation of both UVA and UVB spectrum of different efficacies.

2.1.1. Narrow Band UVB-NBUVB

Narrow band UV (NBUV) of wavelength 311-313 nm can be given to the whole body of vitiligo patients using lamps. Previously, it was considered an effective and safe treatment for hypopigmentation. But, longer exposure to UV radiation may cause skin ageing or skin cancer. In a comparative study conducted by Westerhof and Nieuweboer-Krobotova in 1997 [8], comparing the effect of NBUV and PUVA, the authors reported 46% repigmentation with PUVA, while 67% with NBUV. Due to the better results achieved by NBUV as compared to PUVA, it can be used to a great extent. Combination therapy of NBUV with topical compounds such as afamelanotide was also found to be effective to induce repigmentation in vitiligo patients [9]. Janus kinase (JAK) inhibitors are the promising class of targeted therapy to achieve repigmentation. They have been used in combination with low dose narrow UV-B phototherapy. Tofacitinib and ruxolitinib are the JAK inhibitors that can be taken orally, followed by treatment with narrow band UV-B [10].

Recently, Thu *et al.* [11] have examined the efficacy of narrow band UVB therapy on Vietnamese vitiligo patients. Both segmental and non segmental vitiligo patients were treated with NBUV and found a good response to therapy. The response was significantly good and frequent in the patient with localised non segmental vitiligo than in the patient with generalized non segmental vitiligo. There were no or few adverse effects found in patients. Herpes simplex was developed in one case and mild photo burn was associated with four patients, on adjusting the dose, the burn was completely disappeared.

2.1.2. PUVA Therapy

Oral PUVA therapy is considered as one of the most popular treatments introduced in 1968. It consists of UV radiation of wavelength 320-400 nm and the photosensitizing drugs usually psoralen in the form of 5- methoxypsoralen or 8- methoxypsoralen [12]. The drug can be administered orally 2 hours before light treatment. More frequent side effects associated with these treatment modalities are cutaneous phototoxicities, photo ageing, nausea and the risk of skin cancer [13].

2.1.3. Monochromatic Excimer Light and Laser

Monochromatic excimer light: In this method, a specific wavelength of 308 nm is delivered with xenon chloride gas. This light can be produced by two forms either through an excimer laser that produces a coherent and monochromatic light or the excimer lamp that produces non-coherent light [14]. A double-blind comparative study showed that lamps are time-consuming to deliver a specific dose needed when compared with laser, though there is no difference in response rate found. Additionally, as opposed to NBUVB these forms of treatment may be applied in a more localized way in lesions [15, 16].

Laser: Due to the wide absorption spectrum of melanin, various lasers are effective in the removal of hypopigmented macules including vitiligo, nevus of Ota *etc.* Pulsed dye laser (510 nm), Q-switched ruby laser (694 nm), Q-switched alexandrite laser (755 nm), Nd:YAG laser and Er:YAG laser (1064) are the forms of laser which can remove hypopigmented lesions. They can produce visible green light with a wavelength of 532 nm.

Laser therapy was found to improve the condition of hypopigmentation either alone or in combination with topical treatment. The synergistic effect of the excimer laser with topical immunomodulators has been proved more effective than laser alone [17]. The therapy with an immunomodulator, tacrolimus when combined with 308 nm laser has been reported to be effective for the treatment of hypopigmented scars in adult individuals of Iran [18]. But the combination of 308 nm excimer laser with pimecrolimus has been reported as more effective for the treatment of childhood vitiligo [19]. Li *et al.* [20], have also evaluated the efficiency of 308 nm laser with tacrolimus, pimecrolimus, or halometasome for the treatment of pediatric patients. Patients who received combined therapy of excimer laser and halometasone have found significantly higher rates of repigmentation, even higher than patients who received tacrolimus combined or pimecrolimus combined.

Recently, Eun *et al.* [21] have described the effect of another type of laser, CO_2 fractional laser on idiopathic guttate hypomelanosis (IGH). Fractional Co_2 can remove degenerative melanocytes and keratinocytes from IGH macules in a fractionated manner. Consequently, the lesion would be repigmented by the migration and activation of functional melanocytes of the surrounding normal skin or hair follicles. Previously, Shin *et al.* [22] have reported the effect of fractional Co_2 laser with a high fluence of 100 mJ which requires a week for downtime and local anesthesia. But the work of Eun *et al.* [21] concluded that the low fluence (2-4 mJ) fractional Co_2 laser can also produce therapeutic effects on hypopigmented lesions as compared to those achieved with high fluence.

2.2. Pharmacological Treatment

2.2.1. Topical Corticosteroid

The use of topical corticosteroids in vitiligo treatment is considered as a first-line treatment due to its cost-effectiveness and easy application [23]. The application of corticosteroid topically is appropriate for the treatment of localized vitiligo and hence used on small affected areas particularly elbow, knees, and face. A retrospective study showed that the efficacy of class 3 corticosteroid is higher than that of class 4 corticosteroid. The incidence of atrophy was also observed with class 4 corticosteroid [24].

However, studies recommended the use of high-power corticosteroid but its use is limited to 2-3 months only. So the use of low power corticosteroid is considered in order to minimize the adverse effects. It is also recommended that if there is no clinical response observed in the patient of localized vitiligo after topical corticosteroid application, its use should be discontinued [25].

2.2.2. Immunomodulators

Topical immunomodulators are potent therapeutic agents that work *via* an immunological pathway. It can either suppress or enhance immune and inflammatory responses in the skin. Generally, tacrolimus and pimecrolimus are used as immunomodulators for the treatment of hypopigmented spots including that in vitiligo. The mechanism of action of these drugs involves calcineurin inhibition which results in down-regulation of T-cell reactivity and disturbance in the transcription of proinflammatory cytokine genes which are essential in the pathophysiology of the early immune response [26]. Similarly, prostaglandin E has an immunomodulatory effect on melanocytes and controls their proliferation. It has been used for the treatment of vitiligo and there was significant improvement in vitiligo conditions observed during treatment with the use of topical prostaglandin E [27].

2.3. Surgical Treatment

Vitiligo patients who failed to respond to classical therapies having stable vitiligo are treated with surgical therapy. These methods are generally used for the areas not easy to treat such as elbows, eyelids, knees, and lips. Tissue grafting and cell suspension grafting are the two broad techniques of surgical treatment which consist of the following types:

2.3.1. Tissue Grafting

2.3.1.1. Punch Grafting

Punch grafting is performed by making multiple punches of different sizes on affected areas and then transplanting it with 1-2 mm thickness punch biopsies from the donor area. Better repigmentation with good cosmetic results was observed with punch grafting. Malakar and Dhar [28] observed 90-100% repigmentation rates in around 75% of patients treated with punch graft. The appearance of repigmentation after punch graft was reported as 29 days. The appearance was faster in mucosal followed by segmental, focal, and acrofacial; additionally, quicker in parasternal, infraclavicular areas and lips followed by other areas [29].

An autologous mini punch graft with motorized punches can also be used for stable vitiligo especially on larger areas including difficult sites in a single session which can be effective [30]. There are certain adverse effects found with larger grafts such as cobblestoning which has been corrected with electro fulguration. Studies also proved that punch graft combined with NBUV or topical corticosteroid gives much better results [31, 32].

2.3.1.2.Suction Blister Epidermal Grafting

In this technique, dermo-epidermal separation from the donor site is done by applying constant suction in order to obtain a thin graft and the recipient area is prepared by laser therapy and dermabrasion. A retrospective study showed that more than 75% repigmentation has been achieved in 89% of patients under study [33]. This method offers good therapeutic results but is time-consuming. In a comparative evaluation of punch grafting, suction blister and split-thickness, workers reported that suction blister was more effective than the other two techniques for the removal of hypopigmented scars. It gives cosmetically better results in a shorter duration of time [34].

2.3.1.3. Split Thickness Grafting

Like suction blister grafting, this technique also involves the preparation of the recipient area by dermabrasion followed by a split-thickness graft of the donor area. To obtain a thin skin graft, a dermatome is needed and hence this procedure requires skill and an experienced person to handle dermatome. Sameem *et al.* [35] have described split-thickness grafting as a promising treatment for recalcitrant vitiligo. Ultrathin split-thickness grafting followed by UVB therapy was also reported as an effective treatment option for stable vitiligo. Repigmentation appeared on the second week after ultrathin split grafting followed by UVB therapy and good to excellent results were seen in 90% of the patients [36].

Although it gives good results with 90-100% repigmentation rates as proved by Agrawal and Agrawal [37], there are certain side effects associated with this technique like scarring at normally pigmented donor area and incompatibility of color at recipient area [37, 38].

2.3.2. Epidermal Cell Suspension Grafting

2.3.2.1. Cultured Epidermal Cell Suspension Grafting

This method is definitely beneficial as it increases the number of cells by using the tissue culture technique. Using less donor tissue it can treat larger recipient areas. But this method is costly and require a sophisticated tissue culture laboratory, also the use of certain mitogens in the culture medium raised the question about safety [39]. Non-cultured method on the other hand is much better than cultured method as it is faster and gives better results [40].

2.3.2.2. Non-Cultured Epidermal Cell Suspension Grafting

In this method, the skin fragment is extracted as a biopsy from the donor area. The epidermis is separated from the dermis by treating the skin fragment with trypsin. After consequent steps, suspension of keratinocytes and melanocytes is obtained which is then transplanted to the recipient area. It offers good results with excellent color compatibility at the recipient site [40 - 42].

Although cellular methods have advantages in the surgical management of hypopigmented conditions, such as the requirement of small size donors and efficacy in large hypopigmented macules. But the treatment cost and requirement of special reagents are disadvantages. However, with continued refinement of this technique, they are bound to get extra popularity in the future [43] (Fig. **1**).

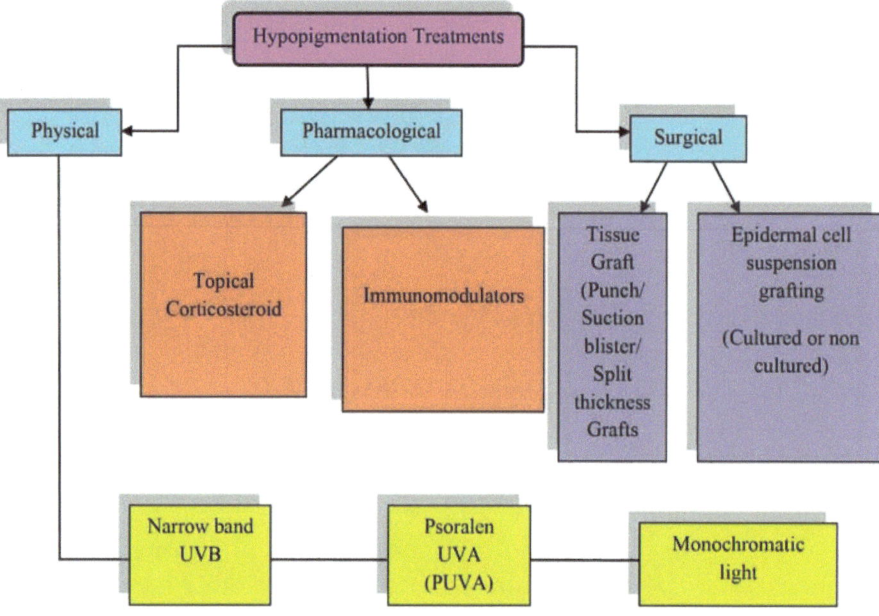

Fig. (1). Overview of the treatments available for hypopigmentation.

3. TREATMENTS AVAILABLE FOR HYPERPIGMENTATION

Treatment for hyperpigmentation appears challenging as no therapy is globally admitted for it, and also the effects of existing agents are variable. Most of the literature regarding treatment for hyperpigmentation contains a small series of patients, so it is not easy to estimate the efficacy of a variety of therapy. Moreover, there are various modalities available but some of them come under growing scrutiny, underscoring the need for research into pathogenesis and treatment. Overall, treatment includes photoprotection, removal of provoking factors, and active pigment reduction with either topical formulations and/or physical methods [44, 45].

3.1. Dermabrasion

Dermabrasion is the technique of superficial removal of upper skin with abrasive tools. Patients suffering from resistant melasma, which was not easy to treat, have successfully been treated with this technique. The use of 16 mm diameter coarse grit diamond fraise in dermabrasion is considered good. Hypertrophic scars or permanent hypopigmentation were found in only 1% of patients but the improvement was found in ninety-seven percent of patients [46]. In other hypoigmentary cases, mild to moderate improvement has been shown with dermabrasion. Histopathological biopsy samples of patients treated with dermabrasion shown to have decreased melanisation and regular distribution of melanosomes [47].

3.2. Chemical Peeling

For the treatment of facial hyperpigmentation, chemical peels can be used either alone or in combination with other regimens. Chemicals that are commonly used in peeling are phenol, trichloroacetic acid, lactic acid, glycolic acid, retinoids, *etc.* In this method, skin damages occur in a controlled manner. Skin gets exfoliated on the application of chemical solution and eventually peels off. As a result, new skin appears with no hyperpigmentary macules. Skin becomes more sensitive to the sun after chemical peeling and hence the use of sunscreen is recommended. Based on the depth of the skin that will exfoliate, chemical peels are of three types: Surface or superficial peel, medium peel and deep peel. Mild acids like alpha hydroxy acids are used in the superficial peel to exfoliate the skin. It only penetrates the outermost layer of the skin. In medium peel, glycolic acid or trichloroacetic acids are used to exfoliate the skin; they penetrate the middle or outer layer of the skin. But deep peels fully penetrate the medium layer of the skin. Among the three types, medium depth peels should be highly recommended and performed with caution and due to the high risk of permanent pigmentary changes, deep peels are not recommended. Even though chemical peels may help to improve hyperpigmentation, they can also cause irritation which leads to hypopigmentation [48].

3.3. Sunscreen

It is evident from various studies that light from both UV and visible range can induce changes in the pigmentation pattern of human skin. UVA and UVB causes increased melanin synthesis, which results in tanning. Hence, protection from the sun is found to be the most essential step which has to be taken to prevent the skin to become hyperpigmented. In order to protect skin from hyperpigmentation, broad-spectrum UVA and UVB protective sunscreen with SPF of at least 30 including a physical block (such as titanium dioxide and zinc oxide) should be recommended [49, 50]. According to Wanitphakdeedecha *et al.* [51], the use of broad-spectrum sunscreen on the first day after skin resurfacing can decrease the incidence of post-inflammatory hyperpigmentation after laser treatment.

3.4. Cosmetic Camouflage

In cosmetic camouflage, cream or powder as makeup is applied to conceal color. Physical blocking opaque sunscreens also have camouflage hyperpigmentation of the face and prevent photoinduced darkening. Many people found that the application of makeup helps to even out the skin tone. Additionally, cosmetic camouflage resolves the psychosocial issues that a skin imperfection is sometimes able to irritate; it allows to rejuvenate its beauty and to return to its own social life [52]. Roberts *et al.* [50] have conducted a single centre clinical trial on females with mild to moderate hyperpigmentation to evaluate the efficacy of multifunctional facial primers. Their study found that those primers were very effective for long term improvement of facial hyperpigmentation when used over a period of 12 weeks.

3.5. Laser Therapy

Laser or light therapy proves a promising and effective treatment for various conditions of hyperpigmentation. Particularly, a longer wavelength is the most often used laser as it can penetrate deeper and can target dermal pigments. Light or laser sources should only be attempted after other regimens have been proven to be ineffective for a particular disease and it should only be used by the experienced physician [54]. As melasma is the common disorder of hyperpigmentation, several treatment modalities have been tried for the management of melasma. Treatment with laser was the most effective one. Q-switched Nd: YAG laser is the most commonly used laser for melasma [55]. Several comparative studies of the effect of different forms of lasers either with laser or other topical application have been done, for the treatment of melasma [56 - 59].

Despite quick and good response with laser, the treatment strategy with the laser has found challenging due to its high risk of damage to surrounding tissues, which results in long-lasting and delayed post-inflammatory hyperpigmentation. So, counselling of patients with regard to side effects and expectations should always be done before any laser therapy [60].

3.6. Topical Treatment

The topical agents used for hyperpigmentation treatment are mostly the chemicals that disrupt the enzymatic processes of pigment production within melanocytes. Agents such as kojic acid, hydroquinone, arbutin, retinoids, *etc.* have been used either alone or in combination with varying degrees of efficacies. The combination of hydroquinone, tretinoin and hydrocortisone called Kligman formulation has been used in the majority of skin lightening creams. Various scientists have successfully tested the modified combination of Kligman formulation which has been now practised in many skin lightening creams. But the regular application of these agents has been found to have various side effects. Hydroquinone is considered the gold standard for hyperpigmentation treatment and has been used for many years but certain side effects including asymptomatic transient erythema, irritation, and exogeneous ochronosis are found to be associated with it [61]. Kojic acid is a known sensitizer which can cause erythema and contact dermatitis. Likewise, arbutin at a higher concentration can cause paradoxical hyperpigmentation [62].

Various national and international brands are claiming that on the application of their creams, the skin will glow in a short span of time. In addition to this, they are claiming that their products are herbal and impart no side effects, so the products are entirely safe. But the fact is that no such thing exist which will glow the skin in a short period of time without the use of certain harmful chemicals such as heavy metals. As reported by Centre for Science and Environment (CSE), around half of the 73 national and international brands of popular cosmetics which were tested, contained a high amount of heavy metals like mercury, cadmium, *etc*. The pollution monitoring lab of CSE had tested some fairness creams and found 44% mercury in it. According to Sunita Narain, Director General CSE, "Mercury is not supposed to be present in cosmetic products". Its mere presence in these products is completely illegal and unlawful [63] (Fig. **2**).

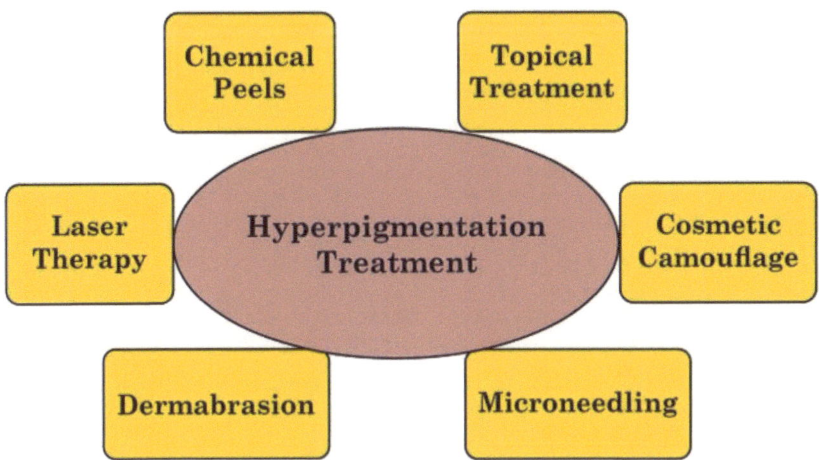

Fig. (2). Overview of the treatments available for hyperpigmentation.

CONCLUSION

Melanin is responsible to impart color to the vertebrate skin but its increased or decreased production and distribution leads to various pigmentary diseases including hyperpigmentation and hypopigmentation. Several treatment modalities have been attempted for the treatment of hypopigmentation including PUVA, NBUVB, laser, tissue grafting, *etc*. Treatment for hyperpigmentation includes a chemical peel, dermabrasion, cosmetic camouflage, topical treatment, *etc*. All the treatment options have different efficacies and can be used as per the condition of the patient.

REFERENCES

[1]   Riley, P.A. Melanin. *Int. J. Biochem. Cell Biol.,* **1997**, *29*(11), 1235-1239.
        [http://dx.doi.org/10.1016/S1357-2725(97)00013-7] [PMID: 9451820]

[2]   Simon, J.D.; Peles, D.; Wakamatsu, K.; Ito, S. Current challenges in understanding melanogenesis: bridging chemistry, biological control, morphology, and function. *Pigment Cell Melanoma Res.,* **2009**, *22*(5), 563-579.
        [http://dx.doi.org/10.1111/j.1755-148X.2009.00610.x] [PMID: 19627559]

[3]   Parveen, N.; Ali, S.A.; Ali, A.S. On the intricacies of facial hyperpigmentation and the use of herbal ingredients as a boon for its treatment: cosmeceutical significance, current challenges and future perspectives. In: *Depigmentation*; In Tech Open publishers: Europe, **2019**; pp. 1-14.
        [http://dx.doi.org/10.5772/60714]

[4]   Parveen, N.; Zaidi, K.U.; Ali, S.A.; Ali, A.S. Microarray as high throughput tool for tyrosinase gene expression analysis. *MOJ Proteomics & Bioinformatics.,* **2017**, *6*(2), 1-4.

[5]   Ali, S.A.; Naaz, I. Current challenges in understanding the story of skin pigmentation — bridging the morpho-anatomical and functional aspects of mammalian melanocytes. in: muscles cells and tissue. In: *Muscles cells and Tissue*; In Tech Open publishers: Europe, **2015**; pp. 261-285.
        [http://dx.doi.org/10.5772/60714]

[6]   Ali, S.A.; Parveen, N.; Ali, A.S. Promoting melanocyte regeneration using different plants and their constituent.*Herbal medicine: Back to the future*; Bentham Science Publishers, **2019**, pp. 247-268.
        [http://dx.doi.org/10.2174/9789811411205119030010]

[7]   Ali, S.A. Recent advances in treatment of skin disorders using herbal products. *J. Skin,* **2017**, *1*(1), 6-7.

[8]   Westerhof, W.; Nieuweboer-Krobotova, L. Treatment of vitiligo with UV-B radiation *vs* topical psoralen plus UV-A. *Arch. Dermatol.,* **1997**, *133*(12), 1525-1528.
        [http://dx.doi.org/10.1001/archderm.1997.03890480045006] [PMID: 9420536]

[9]   Lim, H.W.; Grimes, P.E.; Agbai, O.; Hamzavi, I.; Henderson, M.; Haddican, M.; Linkner, R.V.; Lebwohl, M. Afamelanotide and narrowband UV-B phototherapy for the treatment of vitiligo: a randomized multicenter trial. *JAMA Dermatol.,* **2015**, *151*(1), 42-50.
        [http://dx.doi.org/10.1001/jamadermatol.2014.1875] [PMID: 25230094]

[10]   Kim, S.R.; Heaton, H.; Liu, L.Y.; King, B.A. Rapid repigmentation of vitiligo using tofacitinib plus low-dose, narrowband UV-B phototherapy. *JAMA Dermatol.,* **2018**, *154*(3), 370-371.
        [http://dx.doi.org/10.1001/jamadermatol.2017.5778] [PMID: 29387870]

[11]   Thu, H.D.T.; Hong, N.D.T.; Van, T.N.; Minh, P.P.T.; Van, T.H.; Huu, N.D.; Trong, H.N.; Van, T.C.; Ngoc, T.N.; Hau, K.T.; Gandolfi, M.; Satolli, F.; Feliciani, C.; Tirant, M.; Vojvodic, A.; Lotti, T. The decline of PUVA therapy in vietnam: effective treatment of narrow band uvb in vietnamese vitiligo patients. *Open Access Maced. J. Med. Sci.,* **2019**, *7*(2), 256-258.
        [http://dx.doi.org/10.3889/oamjms.2019.068] [PMID: 30745974]

[12] Lotti, T.; Berti, S.; Moretti, S. Vitiligo therapy. *Expert Opin. Pharmacother.,* **2009**, *10*(17), 2779-2785.
[http://dx.doi.org/10.1517/14656560903357509] [PMID: 19929701]

[13] Pacifico, A.; Leone, G. Photo(chemo)therapy for vitiligo. *Photodermatol. Photoimmunol. Photomed.,*
2011, *27*(5), 261-277.
[http://dx.doi.org/10.1111/j.1600-0781.2011.00606.x] [PMID: 21950634]

[14] Park, K.K.; Liao, W.; Murase, J.E. A review of monochromatic excimer light in vitiligo. *Br. J.
Dermatol.,* **2012**, *167*(3), 468-478.
[http://dx.doi.org/10.1111/j.1365-2133.2012.11008.x] [PMID: 22524428]

[15] Le Duff, F.; Fontas, E.; Giacchero, D.; Sillard, L.; Lacour, J.P.; Ortonne, J.P.; Passeron, T. 308-nm
excimer lamp *vs.* 308-nm excimer laser for treating vitiligo: a randomized study. *Br. J. Dermatol.,*
2010, *163*(1), 188-192.
[http://dx.doi.org/10.1111/j.1365-2133.2010.09778.x] [PMID: 20346025]

[16] Shi, Q.; Li, K.; Fu, J.; Wang, Y.; Ma, C.; Li, Q.; Li, C.; Gao, T. Comparison of the 308-nm excimer
laser with the 308-nm excimer lamp in the treatment of vitiligo--a randomized bilateral comparison
study. *Photodermatol. Photoimmunol. Photomed.,* **2013**, *29*(1), 27-33.
[http://dx.doi.org/10.1111/phpp.12015] [PMID: 23281694]

[17] Passeron, T.; Ostovari, N.; Zakaria, W.; Fontas, E.; Larrouy, J.C.; Lacour, J.P.; Ortonne, J.P. Topical
tacrolimus and the 308-nm excimer laser: a synergistic combination for the treatment of vitiligo. *Arch.
Dermatol.,* **2004**, *140*(9), 1065-1069.
[http://dx.doi.org/10.1001/archderm.140.9.1065] [PMID: 15381545]

[18] Matin, M.; Latifi, S.; Zoufan, N.; Koushki, D.; Mirjafari Daryasari, S.A.; Rahdari, F. The effectiveness
of excimer laser on vitiligo treatment in comparison with a combination therapy of Excimer laser and
tacrolimus in an Iranian population. *J. Cosmet. Laser Ther.,* **2014**, *16*(5), 241-245.
[http://dx.doi.org/10.3109/14764172.2014.946049] [PMID: 25046236]

[19] Hui-Lan, Y.; Xiao-Yan, H.; Jian-Yong, F.; Zong-Rong, L. Combination of 308-nm excimer laser with
topical pimecrolimus for the treatment of childhood vitiligo. *Pediatr. Dermatol.,* **2009**, *26*(3), 354-356.
[http://dx.doi.org/10.1111/j.1525-1470.2009.00914.x] [PMID: 19706108]

[20] Li, L.; Liang, Y.; Hong, J.; Lan, L.; Xiao, H.; Xie, Z. The effectiveness of topical therapy combined
with 308-nm excimer laser on vitiligo compared to excimer laser monotherapy in pediatric patients.
Pediatr. Dermatol., **2019**, *36*(1), e53-e55.
[http://dx.doi.org/10.1111/pde.13726] [PMID: 30520111]

[21] Eun, S.H.; Kwon, H.S.; Ju, H.J.; Jung, H.M.; Lee, J.H.; Oh, S.H.; Bae, J.M. Low-fluence CO_2
fractional laser in the treatment of idiopathic guttate hypomelanosis: A pilot study. *Br. J. Dermatol.,*
2019, *182*(2), 485-486.
[http://dx.doi.org/10.1111/bjd.18427] [PMID: 31396960]

[22] Shin, J.; Kim, M.; Park, S.H.; Oh, S.H. The effect of fractional carbon dioxide lasers on idiopathic
guttate hypomelanosis: a preliminary study. *J. Eur. Acad. Dermatol. Venereol.,* **2013**, *27*(2), e243-
e246.
[http://dx.doi.org/10.1111/j.1468-3083.2012.04597.x] [PMID: 22646755]

[23] Kwinter, J.; Pelletier, J.; Khambalia, A.; Pope, E. High-potency steroid use in children with vitiligo: a
retrospective study. *J. Am. Acad. Dermatol.,* **2007**, *56*(2), 236-241.
[http://dx.doi.org/10.1016/j.jaad.2006.08.017] [PMID: 17224367]

[24] Njoo, M.D.; Spuls, P.I.; Bos, J.D.; Westerhof, W.; Bossuyt, P.M. Nonsurgical repigmentation
therapies in vitiligo. Meta-analysis of the literature. *Arch. Dermatol.,* **1998**, *134*(12), 1532-1540.
[http://dx.doi.org/10.1001/archderm.134.12.1532] [PMID: 9875190]

[25] Falabella, R.; Barona, M.I. Update on skin repigmentation therapies in vitiligo. *Pigment Cell
Melanoma Res.,* **2009**, *22*(1), 42-65.
[http://dx.doi.org/10.1111/j.1755-148X.2008.00528.x] [PMID: 19040503]

[26]   Kostovic, K.; Pasic, A. New treatment modalities for vitiligo: focus on topical immunomodulators. *Drugs,* **2005**, *65*(4), 447-459.
[http://dx.doi.org/10.2165/00003495-200565040-00002] [PMID: 15733009]

[27]   Kapoor, R.; Phiske, M.M.; Jerajani, H.R. Evaluation of safety and efficacy of topical prostaglandin E2 in treatment of vitiligo. *Br. J. Dermatol.,* **2009**, *160*(4), 861-863.
[http://dx.doi.org/10.1111/j.1365-2133.2008.08923.x] [PMID: 19014395]

[28]   Malakar, S.; Dhar, S. Treatment of stable and recalcitrant vitiligo by autologous miniature punch grafting: a prospective study of 1,000 patients. *Dermatology,* **1999**, *198*(2), 133-139.
[http://dx.doi.org/10.1159/000018089] [PMID: 10325459]

[29]   Rajaram, M.; Alagarsamy, S.; Sundarapandiyan, S. Post Punch Graft Appearance of Repigmentation Time in Stable Vitiligo: A Retrospective Study. *Int. J. Sci. Stud.,* **2017**, *5*(5), 81-84.

[30]   Chandrashekar, B.; Madura, C.; Varsha, D. Autologous mini punch grafting: an experience of using motorized power punch in 10 patients. *J. Cutan. Aesthet. Surg.,* **2014**, *7*(1), 42-45.
[http://dx.doi.org/10.4103/0974-2077.129977] [PMID: 24761099]

[31]   Lahiri, K.; Malakar, S.; Sarma, N.; Banerjee, U. Repigmentation of vitiligo with punch grafting and narrow-band UV-B (311 nm)--a prospective study. *Int. J. Dermatol.,* **2006**, *45*(6), 649-655.
[http://dx.doi.org/10.1111/j.1365-4632.2005.02697.x] [PMID: 16796620]

[32]   Saldanha, K.D.; Machado Filho, C.D.; Paschoal, F.M. Action of topical mometasone on the pigmented halos of micrografting in patients with vitiligo. *An. Bras. Dermatol.,* **2012**, *87*(5), 685-690.
[http://dx.doi.org/10.1590/S0365-05962012000500002] [PMID: 23044558]

[33]   Falabella, R. Surgical treatment of vitiligo: why, when and how. *J. Eur. Acad. Dermatol. Venereol.,* **2003**, *17*(5), 518-520.
[http://dx.doi.org/10.1046/j.1468-3083.2003.00718.x] [PMID: 12941084]

[34]   Bali, S.; Singh, M.K.; Soni, A.K. Comparative evaluation of punch grafting, suction blister and split thickness in treatment of stable vitiligo: a prospective study. *Int. J. Contemp. Med. Res.,* **2015**, *4*(4), 77-83.

[35]   Sameem, F.; Sultan, S.J.; Ahmad, Q.M. Split thickness skin grafting in patients with stable vitiligo. *J. Cutan. Aesthet. Surg.,* **2011**, *4*(1), 38-40.
[http://dx.doi.org/10.4103/0974-2077.79189] [PMID: 21572680]

[36]   Majid, I.; Imran, S. Ultrathin split-thickness skin grafting followed by narrowband UVB therapy for stable vitiligo: An effective and cosmetically satisfying treatment option. *Indian J. Dermatol. Venereol. leprosy,* **2012**, *78*(2), 159-164.

[37]   Agrawal, K.; Agrawal, A. Vitiligo: repigmentation with dermabrasion and thin split-thickness skin graft. *Dermatol. Surg.,* **1995**, *21*(4), 295-300.
[http://dx.doi.org/10.1111/j.1524-4725.1995.tb00176.x] [PMID: 7728478]

[38]   Parsad, D.; Gupta, S. Standard guidelines of care for vitiligo surgery. *Indian J. Dermatol. Venereol. Leprol.,* **2008**, *74* Suppl., S37-S45.
[PMID: 18688102]

[39]   Czajkowski, R.; Pokrywczynska, M.; Placek, W.; Zegarska, B.; Tadrowski, T.; Drewa, T. Transplantation of cultured autologous melanocytes: hope or danger? *Cell Transplant.,* **2010**, *19*(5), 639-643.
[http://dx.doi.org/10.3727/096368910X491798] [PMID: 20350353]

[40]   Felsten, L.M.; Alikhan, A.; Petronic-Rosic, V. Vitiligo: a comprehensive overview Part II: treatment options and approach to treatment. *J. Am. Acad. Dermatol.,* **2011**, *65*(3), 493-514.
[http://dx.doi.org/10.1016/j.jaad.2010.10.043] [PMID: 21839316]

[41]   Budania, A.; Parsad, D.; Kanwar, A.J.; Dogra, S. Comparison between autologous noncultured epidermal cell suspension and suction blister epidermal grafting in stable vitiligo: a randomized study.

Br. J. Dermatol., **2012**, *167*(6), 1295-1301.
[http://dx.doi.org/10.1111/bjd.12007] [PMID: 22897617]

[42]   Nahhas, A.F.; Mohammad, T.F.; Hamzavi, I.H. Vitiligo Surgery: Shuffling Melanocytes. *J. Investig. Dermatol. Symp. Proc.,* **2017**, *18*(2), S34-S37.
[http://dx.doi.org/10.1016/j.jisp.2017.01.001] [PMID: 28941491]

[43]   Mysore, V.; Salim, T. Cellular grafts in management of leucoderma. *Indian J. Dermatol.,* **2009**, *54*(2), 142-149.
[http://dx.doi.org/10.4103/0019-5154.53194] [PMID: 20101310]

[44]   Pérez-Bernal, A.; Muñoz-Pérez, M.A.; Camacho, F. Management of facial hyperpigmentation. *Am. J. Clin. Dermatol.,* **2000**, *1*(5), 261-268.
[http://dx.doi.org/10.2165/00128071-200001050-00001] [PMID: 11702317]

[45]   Rigopoulos, D.; Gregoriou, S.; Katsambas, A. Hyperpigmentation and melasma. *J. Cosmet. Dermatol.,* **2007**, *6*(3), 195-202.
[http://dx.doi.org/10.1111/j.1473-2165.2007.00321.x] [PMID: 17760699]

[46]   Kunachak, S.; Leelaudomlipi, P.; Wongwaisayawan, S. Dermabrasion: a curative treatment for melasma. *Aesthetic Plast. Surg.,* **2001**, *25*(2), 114-117.
[http://dx.doi.org/10.1007/s002660010107] [PMID: 11349301]

[47]   El-Domyati, M.; Hosam, W.; Abdel-Azim, E.; Abdel-Wahab, H.; Mohamed, E. Microdermabrasion: a clinical, histometric, and histopathologic study. *J. Cosmet. Dermatol.,* **2016**, *15*(4), 503-513.
[http://dx.doi.org/10.1111/jocd.12252] [PMID: 27357600]

[48]   Cestari, T.; Adjadj, L.; Hux, M.; Shimizu, M.R.; Rives, V.P. Cost-effectiveness of a fixed combination of hydroquinone/tretinoin/fluocinolone cream compared with hydroquinone alone in the treatment of melasma. *J. Drugs Dermatol.,* **2007**, *6*(2), 153-160.
[PMID: 17373174]

[49]   Pathak, M.A.; Riley, F.C.; Fitzpatrick, T.B. Melanogenesis in human skin following exposure to long-wave ultraviolet and visible light. *J. Invest. Dermatol.,* **1962**, *39*, 435-443.
[http://dx.doi.org/10.1038/jid.1962.136] [PMID: 13941837]

[50]   Mahmoud, B.H.; Hexsel, C.L.; Hamzavi, I.H.; Lim, H.W. Effects of visible light on the skin. *Photochem. Photobiol.,* **2008**, *84*(2), 450-462.
[http://dx.doi.org/10.1111/j.1751-1097.2007.00286.x] [PMID: 18248499]

[51]   Wanitphakdeedecha, R.; Phuardchantuk, R.; Manuskiatti, W. The use of sunscreen starting on the first day after ablative fractional skin resurfacing. *J. Eur. Acad. Dermatol. Venereol.,* **2014**, *28*(11), 1522-1528.
[http://dx.doi.org/10.1111/jdv.12332] [PMID: 24320057]

[52]   Sheth, V.M.; Pandya, A.G. Melasma: a comprehensive update: part II. *J. Am. Acad. Dermatol.,* **2011**, *65*(4), 699-714.
[http://dx.doi.org/10.1016/j.jaad.2011.06.001] [PMID: 21920242]

[53]   Roberts, W.E.; Jiang, L.I.; Herndon, J.H., Jr Facial primer provides immediate and long-term improvements in mild-to-moderate facial hyperpigmentation and fine lines associated with photoaging. *Clin. Cosmet. Investig. Dermatol.,* **2015**, *8*, 471-477.
[PMID: 26366102]

[54]   Polder, K.D.; Landau, J.M.; Vergilis-Kalner, I.J.; Goldberg, L.H.; Friedman, P.M.; Bruce, S. Laser eradication of pigmented lesions: a review. *Dermatol. Surg.,* **2011**, *37*(5), 572-595.
[http://dx.doi.org/10.1111/j.1524-4725.2011.01971.x] [PMID: 21492309]

[55]   Shah, S.D.; Aurangabadkar, S.J. Laser Toning in Melasma. *J. Cutan. Aesthet. Surg.,* **2019**, *12*(2), 76-84.
[http://dx.doi.org/10.4103/JCAS.JCAS_179_18] [PMID: 31413475]

[56]   Omi, T.; Yamashita, R.; Kawana, S.; Sato, S.; Naito, Z. Low Fluence Q-Switched Nd: YAG Laser

Toning and Q-Switched Ruby Laser in the Treatment of Melasma:A Comparative Split-Face Ultrastructural Study. *Laser Ther.,* **2012**, *21*(1), 15-4.
[http://dx.doi.org/10.5978/islsm.12-OR-03] [PMID: 24610976]

[57]   Choi, C.P.; Yim, S.M.; Seo, S.H.; Ahn, H.H.; Kye, Y.C.; Choi, J.E. Retrospective analysis of melasma treatment using a dual mode of low-fluence Q-switched and long-pulse Nd:YAG laser *vs.* low-fluence Q-switched Nd:YAG laser monotherapy. *J. Cosmet. Laser Ther.,* **2015**, *17*(1), 2-8.
[http://dx.doi.org/10.3109/14764172.2014.957217] [PMID: 25151913]

[58]   Lee, M.C.; Chang, C.S.; Huang, Y.L.; Chang, S.L.; Chang, C.H.; Lin, Y.F.; Hu, S. Treatment of melasma with mixed parameters of 1,064-nm Q-switched Nd:YAG laser toning and an enhanced effect of ultrasonic application of vitamin C: a split-face study. *Lasers Med. Sci.,* **2015**, *30*(1), 159-163.
[http://dx.doi.org/10.1007/s10103-014-1608-2] [PMID: 25073866]

[59]   Chen, Y.T.; Lin, E.T.; Chang, C.C.; Lin, B.S.; Chiang, H.M.; Huang, Y.H.; Lin, H.Y.; Wang, K.Y.; Chang, T.M. Efficacy and Safety Evaluation of Picosecond Alexandrite Laser with a Diffractive Lens Array for Treatment of Melasma in Asian Patients by VISIA Imaging System. *Photobiomodul Photomed Laser Surg,* **2019**, *37*(9), 559-566.
[http://dx.doi.org/10.1089/photob.2019.4644] [PMID: 31411549]

[60]   Negishi, K.; Akita, H.; Matsunaga, Y. Prospective study of removing solar lentigines in Asians using a novel dual-wavelength and dual-pulse width picosecond laser. *Lasers Surg. Med.,* **2018**, *50*(8), 851-858.
[http://dx.doi.org/10.1002/lsm.22820] [PMID: 29608215]

[61]   Westerhof, W.; Kooyers, T.J. Hydroquinone and its analogues in dermatology - a potential health risk. *J. Cosmet. Dermatol.,* **2005**, *4*(2), 55-59.
[http://dx.doi.org/10.1111/j.1473-2165.2005.40202.x] [PMID: 17166200]

[62]   Draelos, Z.D. Skin lightening preparations and the hydroquinone controversy. *Dermatol. Ther.,* **2007**, *20*(5), 308-313.
[http://dx.doi.org/10.1111/j.1529-8019.2007.00144.x] [PMID: 18045355]

[63]   Narain, S cseindia.org/unregulated-and-unlawful-5293. **2014**.

CHAPTER 7

Natural Product Based Treatment for Hypopigmentation

Abstract: Color of the human skin is primarily due to the presence of pigment melanin, which is produced by the specialized cells called melanocytes. Normal pigmentation is dependent on the normal structure and function of these cells. Irregular lightening of skin lead to hypopigmentary disorder of the skin in which cutaneous and ocular melanocytes are destroyed resulting in loss of pigmentation. Hypopigmentary disorders remained one of the enigmatic issues since the early days of human civilization. Several conventional treatment modalities are available for hypopigmentary disorders; however unsatisfactory results and the indefinite possibility of relapse generally make patients dissatisfied with the treatment. Consequently, the treatment with botanical extracts has better results with less or few side effects. Till date, various plants and their constituents have been tested for their repigmentation activity and results are highly acceptable. In the present chapter, we have emphasized the use of plants and their constituents for the treatment of skin hypopigmentation. Various studies in support of the plant based treatments have also been discussed.

Keywords: Conventional treatment, Disorders, Hypopigmentation, Melanin, Repigmentation.

1. INTRODUCTION

Human skin color is mainly due to the pigment melanin, which is produced inside the specialized cells called melanocytes during the process of melanogenesis. Normal pigmentation is dependent on the normal structure and function of melanocytes. Many factors are involved in proper development of melanocytes from their precursors. Growth, maturation, transferring of melanosomal components, melanin synthesis and then transport and distribution of melanosomes to neighbouring keratinocytes are also the influence of various factors secreted by melanocytes and keratinocytes [1]. Any defect affecting the complex process of skin pigmentation led to the onset of pigmentary disorders, which may be either (a) hyperpigmentary or (b) depigmentary/hypopigmentary [2].

Sharique A. Ali & Naima Parveen

Irregular lightening of skin leading to hypopigmentary disorder of the skin in which cutaneous and ocular melanocytes get selectively destroyed, resulting in pigmentation loss [3]. 1–2% of the population including all races and both sexes are equally affected by it. End of the 19th century witnessed much progress in the field of depigmentary disorders and the term vitiligo vulgaris has been used to describe the malfunctioned process of acquired melanocyte destruction [4]. The pathology of hypopigmentary disorders comprised multiple pathogenic factors, including neural theory, impaired anti-oxidative defenses, genetic predisposition, a link and temporal sequence between oxidative stress and autoimmunity [5].

Hypopigmentary disorder of the skin is characterized by the reduction/complete loss of skin pigmentation. In order to understand the proper mechanism of hypopigmentation, generally three possible theories have been proposed. The first theory is associated with genetic insult that results in melanocytes loss at the time of embryonic development (*e.g.* piebaldism), second theory is about alteration/reduction in production and/or distribution of melanin (*e.g.* oculocutaneous albinism and tinea versicolor) and the third theory is related with the destruction of melanocytes (*e.g.* vitiligo) [6 - 9].

Several conventional treatment modalities, including chemical makeup, topical immunomodulators and corticosteroids, skin grafting, light (UV) and lasers therapy, *etc.*, are available for hypopigmentary disorders. However, unsatisfactory results and the indefinite possibility of relapse generally make patients dissatisfied with the treatment. Additionally, several side effects were found associated with those treatment options such as nausea, headache, vomiting, phototoxicity, photoageing, and hypotrichosis, *etc.* with light/UVB therapy, increase in skin cancer risk, skin atrophy with corticosteroids [10]. To overcome these adverse effects, benefits of natural herbal formulations can be used, which provide opportunities to develop new products as a novel treatment for various hypopigmentory diseases, since medicinal plants are rich sources of bio-active compounds, mostly free from harmful side effects and have been found to be potentially safe and effective skin darkening agents [11, 12].

It became evident from the history of human civilization that human beings have relied on nature for the treatment of disease, as the use of plants or its extract forms the basis of ancient traditional medicines. The advantages of using natural flora as therapeutic agents in treating several ailments are their safety, better patients tolerance, and instead of being inexpensive, they are effective and easily available having a long history of uses [13]. For these reasons, several plants have been investigated for the phytochemical they contained and their role in skin repigmentation. In the present chapter, various studies on plant based treatment of skin hypopigmentation have been discussed.

2. HYPOPIGMENTATION AND ITS RELATED DISORDERS

Hypo pigmentary disorders are characterized by the loss or lack of melanin produced by the melanocytes. These disorders were the most enigmatic issues since the early days of human civilization. Scientific research on hypopigmentary disorders remained relatively basic till the late 1950s as during this period, depigmentation was assumed to be a functional impairment of melanocytes and the concept of melanocyte destruction was not prevalent [14, 15]. Lerner *et al.* [16] demonstrated that destruction and loss of melanocytes occurred in the depigmented area of skin.

Vitiligo, albinism, Vogt-Koyanagi-Harada syndrome, idiopathic guttate hypo-melanosis, pityriasis alba are the variable forms of hypopigmentation. Among all vitiligo, which is also referred as leukoderma, is the most idiopathic disease. The pathologic mechanism of hypopigmentation remained completely obscured until the pioneering work of Hu *et al.* [17], who demonstrated that the affected skin of generalized vitiligo patients generally lacked melanocytes, whereas in the unaffected skin of the same patient, active melanocytes were noticed. These findings led them to propose that the treatment of vitiligo rely totally on either the proliferation of remaining active melanocytes in affected vitiligo skin lesions or immigration or proliferation of functional melanocytes from perilesional area/normal skin [17].

3. CURRENT TREATMENT OPTIONS FOR HYPOPIGMENTATION

Hypopigmentation is the general term used for any type of reduced or absent skin pigmentation. It may be acquired or congenital, generalized or localized and may arise in isolation or be combined with other acquired or congenital disorders. Regardless of a cosmetic disease, the hypopigmentary disorder can be psychologically devastating and stigmatizing [18]. There are varied treatment options for these disorders and depends on the origin or cause of dyspigmentaion. Treatments involve light or laser therapy, use of topical corticosteroids, surgical skin grafting. But among others, PUVA (psoralen and ultraviolet) is the most commonly used treatment and is recommended as the first line therapeutic regimen. For chronic hypopigmentation, treatment involves topical prescription medications. Treatment for the type of hypopigmentation which is unresponsive to medications involves cosmetic tattooing or permanent makeup. Overall depigmentation is the only option for the patients who experience extreme hypopigmentation on over half of their body [19, 20].

4.   CONSEQUENCES OF AVAILABLE TREATMENT FOR HYPOPIGMENTATION

Nevertheless, there are various treatment options available for hypopigmentation, including physical therapies and chemical agents, but not a single option is totally satisfactory. More frequent side effects associated with PUVA and laser treatments are cutaneous phototoxicities, photo ageing, nausea and the risk of skin cancer. Graft rejection is the major drawback of the use of grafting technique for vitiligo patients. The incidence of atrophy was observed with class 4 corticosteroid while used for the treatment of hypopigmentation. Hence, the use of low power corticosteroid should be recommended. Though Q-switched laser induced pigmentation very quickly but various discomforts observed with it [21].

5.   NATURAL PRODUCT BASED TREATMENT FOR HYPOPIGMENTATION

Of late, we have found noteworthy development in the field of research using products of natural origin, demonstrating the rising interest of researchers and pharmaceutical companies in preparing efficacious herbal compounds and their formulations for the treatment of hypopigmentation disorders. Below is the discussion of some of the various plants and their constituents efficiently validated for their repigmentation ability:

5.1. Glycyrrhizin of *Glycyrrhiza Glabra*

Glycyrrhizin is an active ingredient of the plant *Glycyrrhiza Glabra*, recognised as a compound with pharmacological actions. It is a triterpenoid extracted from the rhizomes of the plant *Glycyrrhiza Glabra*. Glycyrrhizin is made up of glucoronic acid (two molecules) and glycyrrhetinic acid (one molecule). The two separate studies based on the effect of glycyrrhizin on melanogenesis have concluded that glycyrrhizin has the potential of melanogenesis stimulation and can be used as a potent agent against hypopigmentary diseases [22, 23]. Out of the two studies, the first study was conducted by Jung *et al.* [22], who have demonstrated that glycyrrhizin upregulates the expression of tyrosinase and tyrosinase related protein- 2 (TRP-2).

In the second study, Lee *et al.* [23] have further explained the involvement of signal transduction pathway in glycyrrhizin induced melanogenesis in B16 melanoma cells. Hence, to clarify the series of events engaged in induced melanogenesis by glycyrrhizin (GR), the authors have treated the B16 cells first with glycyrrhizin and then inhibitors of MEK1, but found that there was no effect on glycyrrhizin induced meanogenesis. On the other hand, when the cells were treated with inhibitors of PKA, it reduces the melanin content. The results of their study imply that mechanism of action of GR induced melanogenesis is *via* cAMP pathway as glycyrrhizin augments the CRE-binding protein (CREB) phosphorylation whereas declines glycogen synthetase kinase 3β and elevates the cAMP production [23].

5.2. *Vigna Angularis* (Adzuki Beans)

Vigna Angularis (Adzuki bean) acts as a remedy for diuretic and used for the treatment of beriberi and dropsy. It is among the most important food material used in East Asian countries. In Japan, it has been used in the production of confectionaries. Itoh and Furuichi [24] have found that synthesis of melanin increases in *in vitro* B16-BL6 melanoma cells on addition of hot water extract of adzuki beans. Tyrosinase assay, protein kinase assay, Rt-PCR and cAMP assay were also performed in order to demystify the exact mechanism of action of water extract (WE) of adzuki beans. It was found that WE activates protein kinase and cAMP pathway of melanogenesis in B16-BL6 cells. They have also performed an *in vivo* study by using C3H-HeJ mice models, in which the mice were given 0.1% (w/v) WE in drinking water and found that WE induced repigmentation in hairs of mice.

5.3. *Piper Methysticum* and *Piper Nigrum*

Five different species of piper were used by Matsuda *et al.* [25] to demonstrate their melanogenesis stimulatory activity on B16 cells; species including *Piper kadsura, Piper longum, Piper betle, Piper cubibain* and *Piper methysticum*. Root extract of *Piper methysticum* was only found to have stimulatory activity on melanogenesis as compared to other species studied. In South Pacific island, roots of *P. methysticum* also known as 'Kava'. It contains a variety of kava lactones like yangonin (+)-kawain, (+)-methysticin, 5, 6-dehydro- kawain and 7,8-epoxyangonin. Among other kavalactones, 7,8-epoxyangonin was observed to have melanogenesis stimulatory activity.

Faas *et al.* [26] have extracted alkaloid piperine and its analogues from *Piper nigrum* and tested their melanogenesis stimulatory potential on thinly pigmented mouse model. It was observed that piperine and its analogues when topically applied with or without UV consecutively for five days (twice a day), there was marked enhancement in pigmentation in test animals. After the end of treatment, histological examination revealed that there was increase in DOPA positive melanocytes in treated mice skin.

5.4. *Vitex Agnus Castus*

It is commonly called as chaste tree which is a shrub that produces aromatic berries. Its berries are used as pepper substitute and as an ingredient in some traditional medicines. It has been reported that chaste berry extract also induce melanin synthesis. An *in vitro* experiment on human melanocytes cell line (R6-NHEM-2) showed that chaste berry extract induces melanogenesis in low concentration also. The effect of chaste berry extract was also tested on twenty women volunteer's skin. Formulation of chaste berry extract using vehicle of palmitic acid, glyceryl stearate, stearic acid, cetyl alcohol and strearyl alcohol *etc* was regularly applied on forearms of volunteers with or without UV. It was found that the tanning response was significantly increased in a dose-dependent manner [27].

5.5. Mediterranean Medicinal Plants

In vitro experiment using B16 melanoma cells performed by Matsuyama *et al.* [28] showed the melanogenesis stimulatory activity of *Capparis spinosa*, *Thymelaea hirsuta* and *Erica multiflora*, which were recognised as Mediterranean plants. They have found that melanin content was significantly increases in a dose dependent manner when treated with *Capparis spinosa* and *Erica multiflora*. DNA microarray and Western blot were also performed to endorse the exact mechanism of melanogenesis induced by plant extracts. Outcomes of their findings confirmed that the extract of *C.spinosa* and *E.multiflora* stimulate melanin synthesis *via* upregulation of tyrosinase expression.

5.6. *Nelumbo Nucifera* (Lotus)

Lotus plant is greatly known for its ornamental values, dietary staple as well as also have medicinal importance in Eastern Asia. Jeaon *et al.* [29] have demonstrated the melanogenesis stimulatory effect of essential oil extracted from nelumbo flower in normal human melanocytes. Through GCMS analysis, it was revealed that essential oil is made up of Palmitic acid methyl ester, linolenic acid methyl ester, palmitolic acid methyl ester. Palmitic acid methyl ester is the essential component which augments the tyrosinase expression and hence plays a crucial role in melanogenesis stimulation.

5.7. Citrus Species

Various species of citrus plant such as *Citrus grandis, C.sinensis, C.paradisi, C.aurantium, C. reticulate, Fructus aurantii* were reported to have an enormous phytochemicals with many pharmacological properties including melanogenic potential. Yoon *et al.* [30] have demonstrated the melanogenic property of nobiletin, a flavonoid isolated from these plants of citrus species in melanoma cells (B16F10). Their results showed that the bioactive compound nobeletin increases the activity of melanogenesis as well as expression of tyrosinase and tyrosinase related protein- 1 (TRP-1) resulted into increase in melanin *via* stimulation of extra cellular signal dependent kinase pathway. Chiang *et al.* [31] have isolated naringenin, the aglycone of naringin from the fruit skin of *Citrus paradise, Citrus grandis, Fructus aaurantii* and *Frustus aaurantii immaturus* to demonstrate their melanogenic effect in melanoma cells (B16F10). They have concluded that naringenin can be used as potential melanogenic agent for hypopigmentation treatment.

Hesperitin, an essential flavonoid extracted from acid hydrolysate of *Citrus reticulate, Citrus sinensis, Citrus aurantium* shown to have melanogenic activity in melanoma cells (B16F10) *via* upregulation of expression of TYR and MITF with an induction of CREB and MAPKs phosphorylation. Results of these findings concluded that hesperetin can be used as melanogenic agent [32].

5.8. Passiflora Species

Park *et al.* [33] have reported that Passiflora species including *Passsiflora edulis, Passiflora incarnate* and *Peganum harmal* has been utilized in oriental medicines for many ailments. Their major bioactive compounds are β-carbolines type alkaloids like harma-lol and harma-line. It was found that these ingredients have melanogenic potential and increases the melanin content, tyrosinase activity, and expression of tyrosinase, tyrosinase related protein1 and tyrosinase protein 2 through P38-MAPK signalling pathway activation in melanoma cells (B16F10) in time and dose dependent manner.

5.9. Seasame Seed and Oil

Seasamin isolated from the seed extract and oil of seasame was found to induce melanin synthesis in melanoma cells (B16) in a dose dependent way *via* stimulation of cAMP pathway without distressing the P38-MAPK resulted in up-regulation of TYRR and MITF expression. Melanogenesis was declined by the inhibitors of PKA but remain unaffected when P38-MAPK and P13K

(Phosphatidylinosiol-3-kinase) inhibitors were used [34]. This confirms the involvement of specific pathway and found that the major pathway of seasamin induced melanin synthesis was cAMP pathway, establishing confirmation of previous studies of Ali *et al.* [35].

5.10. *Pyrostegia Venusta*

This plant is the native of Brazil. The parts of a plant including stems and leaves are utilized in complementary medicines and the flower is used in the treatment of skin white patches. It is a plant with abundant active compounds having known therapeutic potentials. Moreira *et al.* [36] have reported the melanogenesis stimulatory activity of extracts of leaves and flowers of *Pyrostegia venusta* on melanoma cells (B16F10). The leaves and flowers extract was found to contain a significant amount of allantoin. This extract augments the melanin content of melanoma cells in a very little concentration deprived of any effect on the activity of tyrosinase. They have resolved that the leaves and flowers extracts of *P. venusta* can be used as novel melanogenic agent for the management of hypopigmentation.

5.11. *Garcinia Mangostana* (Mangosteen)

It is a native tree of the tropical region of Southern Asia. It has been utilized in Asian countries for its medicinal as well as nutritional values. Using B16F10 melanoma cells, Hamid *et al.* [37] have demonstrated the stimulatory activity of leaf extract of mangosteen on melanogenesis. It was found that the extract of the leaves of mangosteen dose dependently increases the melanin content and tyrosinase activity. Zymograph of tyrosinase was studied to demystify the action of mangosteen extract on increase of activity of intracellular tyrosinase. Through immunoblotting, it was confirmed that mangosteen extract rises the MITF and tyrosinase genes expressions. Their findings suggest that mangosteen extract can be used as promising melanogenic agent.

5.12. *Zanthoxylum Piperitum* and *Sebastiana Schottiana*

Both the plants have common bioactive compound called xanthoxylin, which is a phenolic compound known for its medicinal values. Xanthoxylin was found to have melanogenic property also which was evaluated by Moleephan *et al.* [38] in B16F10 melanoma cells. The confirmation of the involvement of signalling pathways was done by them by means of several cellular and molecular assays. It was observed that xanthoxylin is proficient in stimulation of dendricity and cAMP signalling pathway in B16F10 cells, led to the up-regulation of expression of tyrosinase and MITF. More verification showed that inhibitors of PKA, PKB, PKC and MEK1 reduce mRNA expression of tyrosinase and MITF induced by xanthoxylin which finally leads to decline in melanin content in B16F10 cells. In the light of their findings, the authors have suggested that the main components of the pathway involved in xanthoxylene mediated melanogenesis are cAMP and MEK1.

5.13. Salvia Species

Salvia miltiorrhiza has been extensively used in traditional medicine in China. Chiang *et al*. [39] have demonstrated the melanogenic effect of leaf extract of *S.miltiorrhiza* in B16F10 melanoma cells. Leaf extract of *S.miltiorrhiza* significantly increases the activity of tyrosinase as well as melanin synthesis in a dose dependent manner. Their findings concluded that *S.miltiorrhiza* can be used as repigmenting agent for the treatment of hypopigmentation.

Oleivira *et al*. [40] have explained the melanogenic efficiency of *Salvia officinalis* and its bioactive compound rosmarinic acid (RA) in B16F10 melanoma cells. The extract of *S. officinalis* has been found to bring melanin synthesis in a concentration dependent manner without disturbing free or cellular tyrosinase activity. On the other hand, its active compound rosmarinic acid showed dual nature as in low concentration, it augments the pigment content and TYR activity but in high concentration it showed the opposite effect.

5.14. *Oenanthe Javanica*

O. javanica is a instinctive plant various countries in Asia and found to have enormous amount of bioactive chemicals such as flavonoids, choline, rutamin, γ-fagarine, coumarine. Its melanogenic activity was demonstrated by Kwon and Kim [41], they have tested *O. javanica's* ethanol extract (OJE) containing quercetin and kaempferol in B16F10 cells. Results have showed that the protein expression and tyrosinase activity increases by twelve percent at concentration of 1,000 µg/mL of O. javanica extract. In addition to this, OJE also increases the melanin content in B16F10 cells. In the light of their findings, it was concluded that OJE can be used as a safe repigmentation agent.

5.15. *Larrea Divaricate*

L. divaricate is an evergreen shrub containing lignans as an active compound.

Takekoshi *et al.* [42] showed that a phenolic lignin called nordihydro guaiaretic acid (NDGA) extracted from *L. divaricate* exhibits many pharmacological properties including melanogenic activity. They observed that NDGA induce melanin synthesis in human melanoma cells (HMVII) with increased content of melanin and activity of cellular tyrosinase in time and dose dependent manner. Melanin content of HMVII was found to increase at 20µl concentration after seventh day of treatment. But the mRNA of tyrosinase in HMVII remained unaffected by NDGA treatment. This work puts forward the possibility of treating hypopigmentation diseases including vitiligo using NDGA.

5.16. Chinese Herbs

Lin and Ma [43] have reported the increase in melanogenesis and mushroom tyrosinase activity in mouse melanocytes by the action of Chinese herbs like *Ligustrum lucidum, Fallopia multiflora, Angelica sinensis, etc.* Through HPLC analysis, they have found that Gallic acid, emodin, 2, 3, 5, 4'-tetrahydroxystilbene 2-O-β-D-glucoside (THSG), physcion as major active components of *F. multiflora* (FM). B16F10 melanoma cells on treatment with Extracts of Chinese herbs resulted in eighteen to fifty three percent increase in melanin content in comparison to control without inducing any toxic influence on the viability of cells. The study of Lin and Ma [43] opens an option of utilizing these plants (Chinese herbs) in non-toxic and potent skin or hair blackening cosmetic and/or therapeutic formulation for the treatment of skin hypopigmentation disorders and hair graying.

It is not the termination of the list (Table **1**) as enormous plants and their extracts were scientifically validated through *in vivo* and/or *in vitro* experiments from the past many years for the hunt of developing safe and novel skin darkening ingredients against hypopigmentation [44 - 54] and many more are in pipeline.

Table 1. Scientifically validated plants with their bioactive components having potential of skin repigmentation.

Plant	Active Component	*In vitro/in vivo* Experimental Model	Mode of Action	References
Glycyrrhiza glabra	Glycyrrhizin	B16 melanoma cells	Increases action of TRP-2, Accelerate cAMP pathway Increases level of AP-1 & CREB	[22, 23]

(Table 1) cont.....

Plant	Active Component	*In vitro/in vivo* Experimental Model	Mode of Action	References
Vigna angularis	Hot water adzuki extract	B16-BL6 melanoma cells and C3H/HeJ mice	Increases the production of cAMP, PKA, PKC	[24]
Vitex Agnus Castus (chaste berry)	Casticin Chaste berry extract + acetyl tyrosinase (formulation) +/- UVR	R6-NHEM-2	Increases melanin content	[25]
Citrus paradisi, C. grandis, Fructus aurantii immaturus & Fructus aurantii	Naringenin (4',5,7-trihydroxyflavanone)	B16 melanoma cells	Upregulation of tyrosinase	[27]
Citrus sinensis, C. reticulata, & C. aurantium	Hesperetin	B16/F10 melanoma cells	Increases expression of MAPKs, α-GSK, CREB	[28]
Piper longum, P. kadsura, P. methysticum, P. betle, & P. cubeba	Kavalactones & rhizome extracts	B16 melanoma cells	Increases melanogenesis	[29]
Piper nigrum	Piperine and its 3 analogues + UVA	HRA.HRII-c/+/ Skh hairless pigmented mice	Increases DOPA positive melanocytes and induces repigmentation	[30]
Nelumbo nuficera	Flower essential Oil, Palmitic acid methyl ester	Human skin specimens	Increases expression of MITF-M, TRP-2 TYR	[31]
Capparis spinosa, Erica multiflora	Solvent extract	B16 melanoma cells	Increases Tyrosinase expression and Melanin content	[32]
Passiflora edulis, Passiflora incarnate & Peganum harmala.	β-carbolines alkaloids harmaline & harmalol	B16/F10 melanoma cells	Induce activation of p38 MAPK pathways and increases expression of TYR, TRP1, TRP2	[33]
Garcinia mangostana (Mangosteen)	Leaf extracts	B16/F1 melanoma cells	Increases tyrosinase activity and expression	[36]
Pyrostegia venusta	Crude extracts of leaves and flowers	B16/F10 melanoma cells	Increases melanogenesis	[37]
Salvia miltiorrhiza	Leaf extract	B16/F10 melanoma cells	Increases Tyrosinase and Melanin content	[38]

(Table 1) cont.....

Plant	Active Component	*In vitro/in vivo* Experimental Model	Mode of Action	References
Salvia officinalis	Sage extract or Rosemarinic acid	B16/F10 melanoma cells	Increases Melanin & Tyrosinase activity (low concentration)	[39]
Zanthoxylum piperitum & *Sebastiana schottiana*	Xanthoxylin	B16/F10 melanoma cells	Increases expression of PKA and MITF, increases melanin content	[40]
Oenanthe javanica	Quercetin & kaempferol	B16/F1 melanoma cells	Increases melanin content, Tyrosinase expression, SOD-1, SOD-2, and GSH expression	[41]
Larrea divaricata	Nordihydroguaiaretic acid (NDGA)	Human melanoma cells (HMVII)	Increases melanin content and Tyrosinase activity	[42]
Fallopia multiflora,	2, 3, 5, 4'-Tetrahydroxystilbene 2-O-β-D-glucoside (THSG), gallic acid, physcion, and emodin	B16 melanoma cells	Increases tyrosinase activity	[43]

To understand the action mechanisms of a variety of plants and their active ingredients on pigmentation of skin, our research group is actively working on it in our laboratory. The extracts of various plants including *Psoralea corylifolia* [5, 56], *Piper nigrum* [57], *Chlorophytum borivilianum* [58], *Nigella sativa* [59], *Withania somnifera* [60, 61], *Ficus carica* [62] and *Berberis vulgaris* [63] have been validated by us for their melanogenic activity *via* cholinergic and adrenergic receptors in different animal models such as fishes, reptiles and amphibians. Nevertheless, the exact mechanism by which these plants induces melanogenesis was not fully understood and there is quite substantial scope for the expansion of therapeutic modalities to cure hypopigmentary disorders such as vitiligo.

CONCLUSION

Hypopigmentation is resulted due to deficiency of melanin and/or reduction of melanocytes number. Several treatment modalities including physical, chemical and surgical have been used to overcome the problem of hypopigmentation. But many of them come under increasing scrutiny due to the side effects they imparts. Hence the use of herbal ingredients for the treatment is highly recommended. Keeping in view of the researches carried out on skin darkening efficacy of many plant extracts against hypopigmentation, there are several questions yet to be clear, regarding exact mechanism of action, efficacy in experimental models as many of the stimulators of melanin synthesis have been found to fail in the *in vivo* or clinical tests because either they are not able to penetrate the skin surface or if penetrate, they were ineffective as they loses their biological activity. Hence, novel drug delivery systems are highly recommended and accordingly, there is an urgent need for the implementation of new and potent alternative options to confirm the safety of therapeutic modalities for hypopigmentation.

REFERENCES

[1]　Chiaverini, C.; Beuret, L.; Flori, E.; Busca, R.; Abbe, P.; Bille, K.; Bahadoran, P.; Ortonne, J.P.; Bertolotto, C.; Ballotti, R. Microphthalmia-associated transcription factor regulates RAB27A gene expression and controls melanosome transport. *J. Biol. Chem.,* **2008**, *283*(18), 12635-12642.
[http://dx.doi.org/10.1074/jbc.M800130200] [PMID: 18281284]

[2]　Zaidi, K.U.; Ali, S.A.; Ali, A.; Naaz, I. Natural tyrosinase inhibitors: role of herbals in the treatment of hyperpigmentary disorders. *Mini Rev. Med. Chem.,* **2019**, *19*(10), 796-808.
[http://dx.doi.org/10.2174/1389557519666190116101039] [PMID: 31244414]

[3]　Lerner, A.B. On the etiology of vitiligo and gray hair. *Am. J. Med.,* **1971**, *51*(2), 141-147.
[http://dx.doi.org/10.1016/0002-9343(71)90232-4] [PMID: 5095523]

[4]　Singh, G.; Ansari, Z.; Dwivedi, R.N. Letter: Vitiligo in ancient Indian medicine. *Arch. Dermatol.,* **1974**, *109*(6), 913-917.
[http://dx.doi.org/10.1001/archderm.1974.01630060081032] [PMID: 4598079]

[5]　Khan, N.; Ali, S.A.; Parveen, N. The intricacies of vitiligo with reference to recent updates of treatment modalities. *Eur. J. Pharm. Med. Res.,* **2018**, *5*(2), 187-196.

[6]　Nordlund, J.J. Vitiligo: a review of some facts lesser known about depigmentation. *Indian J. Dermatol.,* **2011**, *56*(2), 180-189.
[http://dx.doi.org/10.4103/0019-5154.80413] [PMID: 21716544]

[7]　Baxter, L.L.; Pavan, W.J. The etiology and molecular genetics of human pigmentation disorders. *Wiley Interdiscip. Rev. Dev. Biol.,* **2013**, *2*(3), 379-392.
[http://dx.doi.org/10.1002/wdev.72] [PMID: 23799582]

[8]　Ali, S.A.; Naaz, I. Current challenges in understanding the story of skin pigmentation: Bridging the morpho-anatomical and functional aspects of mammalian melanocytes. In: *Muscle Cell and Tissue*; Kunihiro, Sakuma, Ed.; InTech Open House: Europe, USA, **2015**.

[9]　Ali, S.A.; Naaz, I. Biochemical aspects of mammalian melanocytes and the emerging role of melanocyte stem cells in dermatological therapies. *Int. J. Health Sci. (Qassim),* **2018**, *12*(1), 69-76.
[PMID: 29623021]

[10]　de Menezes, A.F. Shanmugam, S.; Gomes, I.A.; Oliveira, F.S.; Quintans-Júnior, L.J.; Gurgel Silva, B.S.; Serafini, M.R.; Araújo, A.A.S. (2016). Synthetic Drugs for the treatment of vitiligo: a patent review (2010-2015). *Expert Opin. Ther. Pat.,* **2016**, *29*, 1-13.

[11]　Briskin, D.P. Medicinal plants and phytomedicines. Linking plant biochemistry and physiology to human health. *Plant Physiol.,* **2000**, *124*(2), 507-514.
[http://dx.doi.org/10.1104/pp.124.2.507] [PMID: 11027701]

[12]　Duraipandiyan, V.; Ayyanar, M.; Ignacimuthu, S. Antimicrobial activity of some ethnomedicinal plants used by Paliyar tribe from Tamil Nadu, India. *BMC Complement. Altern. Med.,* **2006**, *6*, 35-41.
[http://dx.doi.org/10.1186/1472-6882-6-35] [PMID: 17042964]

[13]　Zaidi, S.H. Existing indigenous plant resources of Pakistan and their prospects for utilization. *Pakistan Forest J.,* **1998**, *48*(2), 5-8.

[14]   Nordlund, J.J.; Lerner, A.B. Vitiligo. It is important. *Arch. Dermatol.,* **1982**, *118*(1), 5-8.
[http://dx.doi.org/10.1001/archderm.1982.01650130009007] [PMID: 7036910]

[15]   Nordlund, J.J.; Abdel-Malek, Z.A.; Boissy, R.E.; Rheins, L.A. Pigment cell biology: an historical review. *J. Invest. Dermatol.,* **1989**, *92*(4) Suppl., 53S-60S.
[http://dx.doi.org/10.1038/jid.1989.33] [PMID: 2649615]

[16]   Lerner, A.B.; Denton, C.R.; Fitzpatrick, T.B. Clinical and experimental studies with 8-methoxypsoralen in vitiligo. *J. Invest. Dermatol.,* **1953**, *20*(4), 299-314.
[http://dx.doi.org/10.1038/jid.1953.36] [PMID: 13052979]

[17]   Hu, F.; Fosnaugh, R.P.; Lesney, P.F. *In vitro* studies on vitiligo. *J. Invest. Dermatol.,* **1959**, *33*, 267-280.
[http://dx.doi.org/10.1038/jid.1959.150] [PMID: 14403628]

[18]   Sawicki, J.; Siddha, S.; Rosen, C. Vitiligo and associated autoimmune disease: retrospective review of 300 patients. *J. Cutan. Med. Surg.,* **2012**, *16*(4), 261-266.
[http://dx.doi.org/10.1177/120347541201600408] [PMID: 22784519]

[19]   Møller, A.P.; Mousseau, T.A. Albinism and phenotype of barn swallows (*Hirundo rustica*) from Chernobyl. *Evolution,* **2001**, *55*(10), 2097-2104.
[http://dx.doi.org/10.1111/j.0014-3820.2001.tb01324.x] [PMID: 11761068]

[20]   Frisoli, M.L.; Harris, J.E. Vitiligo: Mechanistic insights lead to novel treatments. *J. Allergy Clin. Immunol.,* **2017**, *140*(3), 654-662.
[http://dx.doi.org/10.1016/j.jaci.2017.07.011] [PMID: 28778794]

[21]   Hossani-Madani, A.; Halder, R. Treatment of vitiligo: advantages and disadvantages, indications for use and outcomes. *G. Ital. Dermatol. Venereol.,* **2011**, *146*(5), 373-395.
[PMID: 21956273]

[22]   Jung, G.D.; Yang, J.Y.; Song, E.S.; Par, J.W. Stimulation of melanogenesis by glycyrrhizin in B16 melanoma cells. *Exp. Mol. Med.,* **2001**, *33*(3), 131-135.
[http://dx.doi.org/10.1038/emm.2001.23] [PMID: 11642548]

[23]   Lee, J.; Jung, E.; Park, J.; Jung, K.; Park, E.; Kim, J.; Hong, S.; Park, J.; Park, S.; Lee, S.; Park, D. Glycyrrhizin induces melanogenesis by elevating a cAMP level in b16 melanoma cells. *J. Invest. Dermatol.,* **2005**, *124*(2), 405-411.
[http://dx.doi.org/10.1111/j.0022-202X.2004.23606.x] [PMID: 15675961]

[24]   Itoh, T.; Furuichi, Y. Hot-water extracts from adzuki beans (*Vigna Angularis*) stimulate not only melanogenesis in cultured mouse B16 melanoma cells but also pigmentation of hair color in C3H mice. *Biosci. Biotechnol. Biochem.,* **2005**, *69*(5), 873-882.
[http://dx.doi.org/10.1271/bbb.69.873] [PMID: 15914904]

[25]   Matsuda, H.; Hirata, N.; Kawaguchi, Y.; Naruto, S.; Takata, T.; Oyama, M.; Iinuma, M.; Kubo, M. Melanogenesis stimulation in murine B16 melanoma cells by Kava (*Piper methysticum*) rhizome extract and kavalactones. *Biol. Pharm. Bull.,* **2006**, *29*(4), 834-837.
[http://dx.doi.org/10.1248/bpb.29.834] [PMID: 16595931]

[26]   Faas, L.; Venkatasamy, R.; Hider, R.C.; Young, A.R.; Soumyanath, A. *In vivo* evaluation of piperine and synthetic analogues as potential treatments for vitiligo using a sparsely pigmented mouse model. *Br. J. Dermatol.,* **2008**, *158*(5), 941-950.
[http://dx.doi.org/10.1111/j.1365-2133.2008.08464.x] [PMID: 18284389]

[27]   Schmid, D.; Belser, E.; Zülli, F. Self-tanning Based on Stimulation of Melanin Biosynthesis. *Cosmetics Toiletries,* **2007**, *122*(7), 5562.

[28]   Matsuyama, K.; Miyamae, Y.; Sekii, Y.; Han, J.; Abderrabba, M.; Morio, T.; Shigemori, H.; Isoda, H. Effect of Mediterranean Medicinal Plant Extracts on Melanogenesis Regulation. *J. Arid Land Stud,* **2009**, *19*(1), 387-390.

[29]   Jeon, S.; Kim, N.H.; Koo, B.S.; Kim, J.Y.; Lee, A.Y. Lotus (Nelumbo nuficera) flower essential oil increased melanogenesis in normal human melanocytes. *Exp. Mol. Med.,* **2009**, *41*(7), 517-525.
       [http://dx.doi.org/10.3858/emm.2009.41.7.057] [PMID: 19322028]

[30]   Yoon, H.S.; Lee, S.R.; Ko, H.C.; Choi, S.Y.; Park, J.G.; Kim, J.K.; Kim, S.J. Involvement of extracellular signal-regulated kinase in nobiletin-induced melanogenesis in murine B16/F10 melanoma cells. *Biosci. Biotechnol. Biochem.,* **2007**, *71*(7), 1781-1784.
       [http://dx.doi.org/10.1271/bbb.70088] [PMID: 17617702]

[31]   Chiang, H.M.; Lin, J.W.; Hsiao, P.L.; Tsai, S.Y.; Wen, K.C. Hydrolysates of citrus plants stimulate melanogenesis protecting against UV-induced dermal damage. *Phytother. Res.,* **2010**, *25*(4), 569-76.
       [PMID: 20857432]

[32]   Huang, Y.C.; Liu, K.C.; Chiou, Y.L. Melanogenesis of murine melanoma cells induced by hesperetin, a Citrus hydrolysate-derived flavonoid. *Food Chem. Toxicol.,* **2012**, *50*(3-4), 653-659.
       [http://dx.doi.org/10.1016/j.fct.2012.01.012] [PMID: 22266363]

[33]   Park, S.Y.; Kim, Y.H.; Kim, Y.H.; Park, G.; Lee, S-J. Beta-carboline alkaloids harmaline and harmalol induce melanogenesis through p38 mitogen-activated protein kinase in B16F10 mouse melanoma cells. *BMB Rep.,* **2010**, *43*(12), 824-829.
       [http://dx.doi.org/10.5483/BMBRep.2010.43.12.824] [PMID: 21189160]

[34]   Jiang, Z.; Li, S.; Liu, Y.; Deng, P.; Huang, J.; He, G. Sesamin induces melanogenesis by microphthalmia-associated transcription factor and tyrosinase up-regulation *via* cAMP signaling pathway. *Acta Biochim. Biophys. Sin. (Shanghai),* **2011**, *43*(10), 763-770.
       [http://dx.doi.org/10.1093/abbs/gmr078] [PMID: 21896570]

[35]   Ali, S.A.; Ali, A.S.; Ovais, M.; Belsare, D.K. *In vitro* effect of cyclic AMP on teleost melanophores. *Natl. Acad. Sci. Lett.,* **1985**, *193*, 294-297.

[36]   Moreira, C.G.; Horinouchi, C.D.; Souza-Filho, C.S.; Campos, F.R.; Barison, A.; Cabrini, D.A.; Otuki, M.F. Hyperpigmentant activity of leaves and flowers extracts of *Pyrostegia venusta* on murine B16F10 melanoma. *J. Ethnopharmacol.,* **2012**, *141*(3), 1005-1011.
       [http://dx.doi.org/10.1016/j.jep.2012.03.047] [PMID: 22504061]

[37]   Hamid, M.A.; Sarmidi, M.R.; Park, C.S. Mangosteen leaf extract increases melanogenesis in B16F1 melanoma cells by stimulating tyrosinase activity *in vitro* and by up-regulating tyrosinase gene expression. *Int. J. Mol. Med.,* **2012**, *29*(2), 209-217.
       [PMID: 22089762]

[38]   Moleephana, W.; Wittayalertpanyab, S.; Ruangrungsic, N.; Limpanasithikul, W. Effect of xanthoxylin on melanin content and melanogenic protein expression in B16F10 melanoma. *Asian Biomed.,* **2012**, *6*(3), 413-422.

[39]   Chiang, S.H.; Chen, Y.S.; Hung, M.S.; Lee, S.M.; Lin, C.C. The enhancement effect of *Salvia miltiorrhiza* on melanin production of B16F10 melanoma cells. *J. Med. Plants Res.,* **2012**, *6*(26), 4338-4342.

[40]   Oliveira, K.B.; Palú, É.; Weffort-Santos, A.M.; Oliveira, B.H. Influence of rosmarinic acid and *Salvia officinalis* extracts on melanogenesis of B16F10 cells. Brazil. *J. Pharmacol.,* **2013**, *23*(2), 249-258.

[41]   Kwon, E.J.; Kim, M.M. Effect of *Oenanthe javanica* ethanolic extracts on antioxidant activity and melanogenesis in melanoma cells. *J. Life Sci.,* **2013**, *23*(12), 1428-1435.
       [http://dx.doi.org/10.5352/JLS.2013.23.12.1428]

[42]   Takekoshi, S.; Nagata, H.; Kitatani, K. Stimulation of melanogenesis by nordihydroguaiaretic Acid in human melanoma cells. *Acta Histochem. Cytochem.,* **2014**, *47*(5), 203-210.
       [http://dx.doi.org/10.1267/ahc.14033] [PMID: 25861126]

[43]   Lin, S.H.; Ma, L.J. Effects of chinese herbal extracts on tyrosinase activity and melanogenesis. *Nat. Prod. Chem. Res.,* **2015**, *3*(4), 1-4.

[44]   Chun, H.J.; Jeong, S.I.; Woo, W.H.; Kim, I.K. Effect of Ikarisoside A Isolated from Epimedium Koreanum on Melanogenesis. *Bull. Korean Chem. Soc.,* **2001,** *22*(10), 1159-1162.

[45]   Matsuda, H.; Hirata, N.; Kawaguchi, Y.; Yamazaki, M.; Naruto, S.; Shibano, M.; Taniguchi, M.; Baba, K.; Kubo, M. Melanogenesis stimulation in murine b16 melanoma cells by umberiferae plant extracts and their coumarin constituents. *Biol. Pharm. Bull.,* **2005,** *28*(7), 1229-1233.
[http://dx.doi.org/10.1248/bpb.28.1229] [PMID: 15997104]

[46]   Guan, S.; Su, W.; Wang, N.; Li, P.; Wang, Y. A potent tyrosinase activator from Radix *Polygoni multiflori* and its melanogenesis stimulatory effect in B16 melanoma cells. *Phytother. Res.,* **2008,** *22*(5), 660-663.
[http://dx.doi.org/10.1002/ptr.2358] [PMID: 18389468]

[47]   Datta, K.; Singh, A.T.; Mukherjee, A.; Bhat, B.; Ramesh, B.; Burman, A.C. *Eclipta alba* extract with potential for hair growth promoting activity. *J. Ethnopharmacol.,* **2009,** *124*(3), 450-456.
[http://dx.doi.org/10.1016/j.jep.2009.05.023] [PMID: 19481595]

[48]   Mohamed, A.A.K.; El-Saman, S.F.M. Light and electron microscopic studies of the effect of combined topical calcipotriol and PUVA therapy on patients with vitiligo. *Egypt. J. Histol.,* **2011,** *34,* 15-27.
[http://dx.doi.org/10.1097/01.EHX.0000394884.67992.01]

[49]   Kumar, N.; Rungseevijitprapa, W.; Narkkhong, N.A.; Suttajit, M.; Chaiyasut, C. 5α-reductase inhibition and hair growth promotion of some Thai plants traditionally used for hair treatment. *J. Ethnopharmacol.,* **2012,** *139*(3), 765-771.
[http://dx.doi.org/10.1016/j.jep.2011.12.010] [PMID: 22178180]

[50]   Villareal, M.O.; Han, J.; Matsuyama, K.; Sekii, Y.; Smaoui, A.; Shigemori, H.; Isoda, H. Lupenone from *Erica multiflora* leaf extract stimulates melanogenesis in B16 murine melanoma cells through the inhibition of ERK1/2 activation. *Planta Med.,* **2013,** *79*(3-4), 236-243.
[http://dx.doi.org/10.1055/s-0032-1328189] [PMID: 23408272]

[51]   Kim, H.J.; Kim, I.S.; Dong, Y.; Lee, I.S.; Kim, J.S.; Kim, J.S.; Woo, J.T.; Cha, B.Y. Melanogenesis-inducing effect of cirsimaritin through increases in microphthalmia-associated transcription factor and tyrosinase expression. *Int. J. Mol. Sci.,* **2015,** *16*(4), 8772-8788.
[http://dx.doi.org/10.3390/ijms16048772] [PMID: 25903150]

[52]   An, Y.A.; Hwang, J.Y.; Lee, J.S.; Kim, Y.C. Cornus officinalis Methanol extract upregulates melanogenesis in melan-a cells. *Toxicol. Res.,* **2015,** *31*(2), 165-172.
[http://dx.doi.org/10.5487/TR.2015.31.2.165] [PMID: 26191383]

[53]   Yao, C.; Jin, C.L.; Oh, I.G. Park, Chi-Hyun.; Chung, J.H. *Melia azadarach* extract stimulates melanogenesis through increase in tyrosinase-related protein1 (TRP1) expression in B16 mouse melanoma cells. *Int. J. Mol. Med.,* **2015,** *35*(6), 1761-1766. a
[http://dx.doi.org/10.3892/ijmm.2015.2182] [PMID: 25872655]

[54]   Yao, C.; Jin, C.L.; Oh, J.H.; Oh, I.G.; Park, C.H.; Chung, J.H. *Ardisia crenata* extract stimulates melanogenesis in B16F10 melanoma cells through inhibiting ERK1/2 and Akt activation. *Mol. Med. Rep.,* **2015,** *11*(1), 653-657. b
[http://dx.doi.org/10.3892/mmr.2014.2697] [PMID: 25333888]

[55]   Sultan, T.; Ali, S.A. *Psoralea corylifolia* extracts stimulate cholinergic-like psoralen receptors of tadpole-tail melanophores, leading to skin darkening. *J. Recept. Signal Transduct. Res.,* **2011,** *31*(1), 39-44.
[http://dx.doi.org/10.3109/10799893.2010.508164] [PMID: 20863173]

[56]   Ali, S.A.; Sultan, T.; Galgut, J.M.; Sharma, R.; Meitei, K.V.; Ali, A.S. *In vitro* responses of fish melanophores to lyophilized extracts of *Psoralea corylifolia* seeds and pure psoralen. *Pharm. Biol.,* **2011,** *49*(4), 422-427.
[http://dx.doi.org/10.3109/13880209.2010.521164] [PMID: 21391886]

[57]   Sajid, M.; Ali, S.A. Mediation of cholino-piperine like receptors by extracts of *Piper nigrum* induces melanin dispersion in *Rana tigerina* tadpole melanophores. *J. Recept. Signal Transduct. Res.,* **2011,** *31*(4), 286-290.
[http://dx.doi.org/10.3109/10799893.2011.583254] [PMID: 21663558]

[58]   Chaudhari, S.A.; Peter, J.; Galgut, J.M.; Ali, S.A. Melanin inhibitory and melanin stimulatory effects of extracts of *Chlorophytum tuberosum* and *Chlorophytum borivilianum* on isolated fish scale melanophores. *Afr. J. Pharm. Pharmacol.,* **2012,** *6*(12), 919-923.

[59]   Ali, S.A.; Meitei, K.V. *Nigella sativa* seed extract and its bioactive compound thymoquinone: the new melanogens causing hyperpigmentation in the wall lizard melanophores. *J. Pharm. Pharmacol.,* **2011,** *63*(5), 741-746. a
[http://dx.doi.org/10.1111/j.2042-7158.2011.01271.x] [PMID: 21492177]

[60]   Ali, S.A.; Meitei, K.V. On the action and mechanism of withaferinA from *Withania somnifera* a novel and potent melanin dispersing agent in frog melanophores. *J. Recep. Signal Transduct.,* **2011,** *31*(5), 367-373. b

[61]   Ali, S.A.; Meitei, K.V. *Withania somnifera* root extracts induce skin darkening in wall lizard melanophores *via* stimulation of cholinergic receptors. *Nat. Prod. Res.,* **2012,** *26*(17), 1645-1648.
[http://dx.doi.org/10.1080/14786419.2011.589053] [PMID: 21950559]

[62]   Meitei, K.V.; Ali, S.A. Fig leaf extract and its bioactive compound psoralen induces skin darkening effect in reptilian melanophores *via* cholinergic receptor stimulation. *In Vitro Cell. Dev. Biol. Anim.,* **2012,** *48*(6), 335-339.
[http://dx.doi.org/10.1007/s11626-012-9521-0] [PMID: 22706602]

[63]   Ali, S.A.; Naaz, I.; Choudhary, R.K. Berberine-induced pigment dispersion in *Bufo melanostictus* melanophores by stimulation of beta-2 adrenergic receptors. *J. Recept. Signal Transduct. Res.,* **2014,** *34*(1), 15-20.
[http://dx.doi.org/10.3109/10799893.2013.843193] [PMID: 24099619]

CHAPTER 8

Natural Product Based Treatment for Hyperpigmentation

Abstract: Melanin is responsible to impart color to the skin as well as to provide protection from harmful UV radiation. But it's excess production and distribution leads to hyperpigmentation and its related disorders. Several treatment strategies have been used to treat the problem of hyperpigmentation, including chemical peeling, dermabrasion, laser, topical treatment, *etc*. But skin burn, dyspigmentation, acne, swelling, pain *etc*. are some of the after effects found associated with these treatment options. To keep in view of the side effects of current treatment modalities and in order to get rid of the problem of hyperpigmentation, scientists were focussed on traditional system of treatment in which the skin treatment was done by natural products, which are without toxicological implications. Hence, various medicinal plants and their constituents having few or no risk of side effects have been tested for their efficacies to treat disorders of hyperpigmentation. In the present chapter, we have discussed some of those plants and their active ingredients which have been successfully used for the treatment of hyperpigmentation.

Keywords: Hyperpigmentation, Medicinal plants, Melanin, Natural products, Side effects.

1. INTRODUCTION

Pigment melanin is the biopolymer responsible to impart color to the integument, hair, and eyes as well as protects the skin from harmful ultraviolet radiation. Melanogenesis is the complex process of producing melanin inside the specialized organelles of melanocytes [1]. Even though melanin defends the skin from UV radiation but its extra production results in hyperpigmentation and its related disorders [2]. The common diseases of hyperpigmentation includes post inflammatory disorders, solar lentigens, ephelides, melasma, *etc*. Due to hyperpigmentation spots on the face, skin become imperfect which ultimately causes psychological issues in patients and takes them away from their social lives. The insights of people for lighter skin as being attractive and healthy in addition to rising demand of hyperpigmentation problem aggravate vast interest pharmaceutically and cosmeceutically [3].

Today, the problem of hyperpigmentation is the common and growing concern to the dermatologists. As there is no treatment for hyperpigmentation is universally accepted and also the efficacy of various lightening agents are different [4]. Most of the reports concerning the management of disease involve small number of patients. Thus, it becomes challenging to assess the effect of variety of therapy [5]. Additionally, there are several options but many of them come under emergent inspection, forcing the research into pathogenesis and treatment. Cosmetic camouflage, chemical peeling, dermabrasion, use of sunscreen, laser therapy and topical treatment are the different strategies used to treat hyperpigmentation. Despite being very effective and fast, these treatment strategies on their long term usage causes various side effects. Some of those side effects include swelling, pain, acne, persistent erythema, dyspigmentation, herpes recurrence, and allergic reactions [6].

In contrast to the state of affairs with these treatment modalities, we have other side of treatment with compounds of natural origin like plants that are currently getting importance due to their reduced cost, easy to use and are believed to be free from risk of handling them and hardly pollute the environment [7]. Subsequently, scientists have designed such dermatological formulations containing bioactive compounds of strictly natural origin to protect the skin from harmful exogenous and endogenous agents. Various chemical reactions involving many enzymes are engaged in melanin synthesis. Hence, there is a huge range of mechanisms against which to screen for pigmentation control agents [8]. The active compounds isolated from various plants inhibit melanin synthesis *via* different mechanisms such as inhibition of tyrosinase activity, inhibition of expression of tyrosinase and related proteins, inhibition of melanosome transfer to keratinocytes, *etc.* [9].

Since, there is enormous flora available on earth that has many therapeutic properties, they are used for the management of various life style diseases. Accordingly, plants and their active ingredients are used for the treatment of hyperpigmentation *via* different mechanisms of action. Various plants and their studies on hyperpigmentation treatment by different scientists have been discussed in the present chapter.

2. HYPERPIGMENTATION AND ITS RELATED DISORDERS

The synthesis and distribution of melanin depend on the specialized cells called melanocytes through the process of melanogenesis. It involves various steps from the development of an embryo, synthesis of melanin, and transfer of melanosomes to neighbouring keratinocytes [10]. The significance of these steps and their mechanisms is evident in pigmentation defects in the form of hyperpigmentation and hypopigmentation [11]. When the skin exposes to UV radiation or other endo or exogenous allergen causes formation of inflammatory mediators, erythema, excess production of melanin which ultimately results in pigmentation disorder called hyperpigmentation [12].

Post inflammatory hyperpigmentation, maturational dyschromia, melasma, solar lentigines, ephelides, lichen planus pigmentosus are the various diseases of hyperpigmentation. Melasma is the common disorders of hyperpigmentation affecting thousands of the individual worldwide and about 90% are females. Melasma is also known as 'the mask of pregnancy' because the condition is often associated with pregnant women. Hyperpigmentation refers to the darkening of the skin in patches. Size and symmetry of the hyperpigmented patches or macules are different in different forms of hyperpigmentation diseases. Skin hyperpigmentation started from the sun exposed areas of the body including face, neck, trunk, forehead, *etc.* [13].

3. AVAILABLE TREATMENT MODALITIES FOR HYPERPIGMENTATION

Treatment for hyperpigmentation seems to be challenging as there is no completely satisfactory treatment available and also the existing depigmentation agents have different efficacy. Generally, the target of treatment includes reduction of pigment either topically or physically, photoprotection, elimination of provoking factors [14, 15]. Treatments for hyperpigmentation include use of sunscreen, chemical peel, cosmetic camouflage, dermabrasion, topical treatment, treatment with laser, *etc.* In chemical peeling, a chemical solution is applied to the skin which makes it exfoliate and ultimately peel off. Cosmetic camouflage is the application of makeup including cream, powder to conceal colour. Dermabrasion is the process of removal of upper skin, non chemically with abrasive tools. Laser of shorter or longer wavelength can also be used to treat pigmented skin. Topical treatment includes the application of different chemical agents such as kojic acid, hydroquinone, arbutin, *etc.* which can be used either alone or in combination.

4. LIMITATIONS OF CURRENT TREATMENT OPTIONS

At present, there are various treatment strategies for hyperpigmentation available such as physical therapy and chemical analogues, but none of them are totally acceptable. Hydroquinone, kojic acid, arbuin are the traditional topical agents with extremely high efficiency, but when they are used for a long time it causes various side effects. Chemical peeling, dermabrasion, laser therapy, cosmetic camouflage are the treatment modalities which imparts several after effects including swelling, pain, persistent erythema, herpes recurrence, dyspigmentation, acne, *etc.* [16, 17].

It was observed that the patients exhibited itching, swelling, and erythema on their whole face when treated with tritenoin containing chemical peel [18]. There is a risk of damage to the surrounding tissues when treated with laser therapy [18]. Although the use of 50 plus sun protection factor (SPF) may defend the skin from suntan but when it is used for a long term, it causes reduction in vitamin D production of skin which is needed for the health of bones and ultimately increases the risk of osteoporosis [19].

5. NATURAL PRODUCT BASED TREATMENT FOR HYPERPIGMENTATION

As there are various disadvantages of current modalities of treatment for hyperpigmentation, the dermatologists as well as scientists of the world are now searching for such treatment which will be safe with less or no side effects and at the same time not contaminating the environment. Therefore, the application of plants and their active biocompounds for skin hyperpigmentation treatment is attaining wide interest as these compounds are safe and mild in comparison to synthetic ingredients. Various formulations having active ingredients of natural origin are designed and developed to prevent cutaneous hyperpigmentation. The main objective of using natural compounds is to minimize hyperpigmentation without causing irritation or undesirable dyspigmentation in skin [9].

Many enzymes and processes are involved in melanogenesis therefore there are numerous targets or mechanisms which need to be screened for skin pigmentation control agents. The bioactive ingredients isolated from various plants have been found to inhibit melanogenesis without melanocyte toxicity by several mechanisms such as inhibition of activity of tyrosinase, inhibition of expression of tyrosinase and its related proteins and/or inhibition of melanosome transfer to keratinocytes.

5.1. Inhibition of Tyrosinase Activity

As the enzyme tyrosinase is the key enzyme of melanogenesis, its inhibitors seeks the interest of scientists to check the undesirable production of melanin. There are numerous agents of natural origin which are acting through interfering in the pathways of melanogenesis by inhibiting the activity of tyrosinase [20].

Various aldehydes and other derivatives isolated from plants were found to have tyrosinase inhibitory activity such as cuminaldehyde and cumic acid [21], (2E)-alkenals [22], 2-hydroxy-4-methoxybenzaldehyde [22], transcinnamaldehyde [23], 3,4-dihydroxycinnamic acid and 4-hydroxy-3-methoxycinnamic acid [24], anisaldehyde [25]. Aldehyde group is known to react with biologically essential nucleophilic groups including hydroxyl, amino, sulfhydryl, *etc.*, so its inhibitory activity is due to the formation of Schiff base with the primary amino group of tyrosinase. In cuminaldehyde the electron donar groups, including isopropyl and methoxy group at the para position, provides stability to the Schiff base at the active site of tyrosinase through inductive effect [21].

Plenty of work has been done for the identification and characterization of tyrosinase inhibitors from natural sources and for the establishment of the relationship between their inhibitory activity and structure. Flavonoids isolated from plants can inhibit tyrosinase activity due to their capability of chelating the copper ion present in the active site of tyrosinase. Flavonoids such as kaempferol, quercetin, kurarinone, kushnol F with strong tyrosinase activity has been isolated from various plants [26 - 29]. P-coumaric acid extracted from Panax ginseng leaves has been found to inhibit L-tyrosine oxidation [30]. It inhibits monophenolase as well as diphenolase activities and a polar hydroxyl group present at para position of p- coumaric acid increases monophenolase activity. The tyrosinase inhibitory effect of p-coumaric acid was also recently described by Boo [31]. Potent tyrosinase inhibitory activity was also shown by oxyresveratrol due to the presence of polar hydroxyl groups in the ring [32]. Badria and el Gayyar [33] have reported that flavonoids containing keto group acquire potent tyrosinase inhibitory activity. It can be explained in terms of similarity between the dihydroxyphenyl group in L-DOPA and keto group in flavonoids. Results of the study revealed another type of flavonoids isolated from a natural source as a tyrosinase inhibitor.

1,2,3,4,6-PentaO-galloyl-d-glucose (PGG) isolated from *G. Rhois* [34] has a strong tyrosinase inhibitory activity, however, this is not reliable with previous reports which showed that the tyrosinase inhibitory activity of aromatic carboxylic acids decreases with hydroxylation, esterification, and methylation of the benzene ring [35, 36]. The three main components including gallocatechin gallate, epicatechin gallate and epigallocatechin gallate extracted from leaves of green tea and their tyrosinase inhibitory effect were assessed and described green tea as a strong inhibitor of tyrosinase. The study indicates that the flavon-3-ol skeleton with a galloyl moiety at the 3-position is the reason for the inhibition of tyrosinase activity. Through kinetic studies, it was found that these compounds inhibit tyrosinase in a competitive manner [37]. Taxifolin, belongs to the class of flavonoids, was isolated from the sprouts of *Polygonum hydropiper* and have been shown potent tyrosinase inhibitory activity [38].

Hridya *et al.* [39] and Hridya *et al.* [40] showed that santalin extracted from *Pterocarpus santalinus* and brazilein isolated from *Caesalpinia sappan* was found to reversibly inhibit tyrosinase in a dose dependent mixed type manner. In order to find out compounds with tyrosinase inhibitory activity from *Sophora flavescens*, Kim *et al.* [41] have extracted five flavonoids, including 8-prenylkaempferol, kushenol A, kushenol C, 8- prenylnaringenin, formononetin. Their results found that among the five isolated compounds, kushenol A and 8-prenylnaringenin exhibited potent tyrosinase inhibitory activity which was further confirmed by molecular docking. Recently Lee *et al.* [42] have isolated and characterized 17 compounds from *Achillea alpine* and among all, compound 15 was found to suppress the intracellular tyrosinase activity. Similarly, Tang *et al.* [43] have purified and characterized polysaccharides from chestnut (*Castanea mollissima*). Ultrasound extracted polysaccharide fractions 1 and 2 showed inhibition of intracellular tyrosinase activity, monosaccharide composition of both polysaccharides was glucose, fructose, mannose, galactose, arabinose, xylose, rhamnose with different proportion. Three hydroxycinnamic acids including p-coumaric acid, caffeic acid, rosmarinic acid have been isolated by Crespo *et al.* [44] from *Lepechinia meyenii* and found that they have a strong affinity for tyrosinase which inhibit its activity.

5.2. Inhibition of Expression of Tyrosinase and its Related Proteins

Many compounds of natural origin have been tested and aimed at inhibiting the production and expression of enzymes such as tyrosinase, tyrosinase related protein-1 (TRP-1), and tyrosinase related protein-2 (TRP-2), which are involved in rate limiting steps of melanin synthesis pathway.

Rho *et al.* [45] have isolated three active compounds incuding N-feruloyserotonin, N-(p-coumaroyl) serotonin and acacetin from *Carthamus tinctorius*, which were found to inhibit the melanin synthesis in B16 melanoma cells by inhibiting the expression of TYR, TRP-1 and TRP-2. Cho *et al.* [46] have isolated macelignan from the plant *Myristica fragrans*. It has shown melanogenesis inhibition activity *via* decreased expression of TYR, TRP-1 and TRP-2 in melan-a murine melanocytes. Macelignan effectively inhibits melanin synthesis and could be used as a new skin whitening agent [46]. Calycosin isolated from the roots of *Astragalus membranaceus* has been found to reduce the expression and the activity of tyrosinase, so it might be used for skin lightening [47]. Fuji *et al.* [48] have demonstrated that quercetin isolated from rose hip (*Rosa canica*) has antimelanogenic effect by suppressing the expression of melanogenic enzymes, including tyrosinase.

Lee *et al.* [49] isolated panduratin A from *Kaempferia pandulata* to assess its inhibitory activity against melanin biosynthesis. Panduratin A has shown decreased expression of tyrosinase, TRP-1, TRP-2 as confirmed by Western blot analysis. Similarly, piceid isolated from *Polygonum cuspidatum* inhibits melanogenesis by decreasing the expression of tyrosinase [50]. Studies of Lee *et al.* [51] showed that curcumin decreased the expression of melanogenesis related protein such as TYR, TRP-1 and TRP-2 and MITF in alpha melanocyte stimulating hormone (MSH) stimulated B16F10 melanoma cells. Acteoside is the glycoside isolated from the leaves of *Rehmannia glutinosa*, which has inhibitory activity on melanin synthesis by reducing the levels of tyrosinase, TRP-1, TRP-2 and MITF [52]. Kim *et al.* [53] have isolated octaphlorethol A from *Ishige foliacae*, which markedly inhibited melanin synthesis and decreased tyrosinase, TRP-1, TRP-2 and MITF expressions. Similarly, doscin was chemically isolated and explored for its effect on melanogenesis. Immuno blot analysis revealed that it reduced the expression of tyrosinase, TRP-1 and TRP-2, resulting in inhibition of intracellular production of melanin [54].

Panax ginseng has been used as a medicinal plant which has many ginsenoside with several therapeutic potentials including inhibitory effect on melanin synthesis. Floralginsenoside (FGA), ginsenoside Re (GR), ginsenoside Rd (GRD) extracted from *P.ginseng*. Floralginsenoside (FGA) was found to have more inhibitory effect on melanin synthesis *via* decreased expression of MITF in a dose dependent way. Additonally, it was observed that FGA also induced extracellular signal regulated kinase phosphorylation level in melan-a-cells [55]. Liu *et al.* [56] have recently isolated another active compound, vanillic acid from *Panax ginseng* root. Vanillc acid has also been shown to decrease the expression of micropthalmia associated transcription factor and hence inhibit melanin biosynthesis. The depigmenting activity of 10-hydroxy-2-decenoic acid (10-HAD) isolated from royal jelly of *Apis mellifera* was evaluated by Peng *et al.* [57]. They have observed that 10-HAD reduced melanogenesis *via* inhibiting TYR, TRP-1, TRP-2 and MITF expression in B16F1 melanoma cells.

The findings of Ko *et al.* [58] showed that n-hexane fraction of *Sageretia thea* downregulated melanogenesis *via* decreased expression of TYR, TRP-1, TRP-2 and MITF. Methyl linoleate and methyl linolenate were the active ingredients identified by gas chromatography mass spectrometry (GC-MS), which was responsible for melanogenesis inhibition. Lim *et al.* [59] have investigated the melanogenic suppression effect of dehydroglyasperin C (DGC), an active component from *Glycyrrhiza uralensis*. DGC decreased intracellular activity of tyrosinase as well as expression of melanin synthesis related proteins including tyrosinase, TRP1 and TRP2. Sargaquinoic acid isolated from the ethanolic extract of *Sargassum serratifolium* ameliorated hyperpigmentation *via* cAMP and ERK mediated downregulation of MITF in B16F10 melanoma cells. Similarly, sargaquinoic acid attenuated melanin synthesis by inhibiting the expression of tyrosinase, TRP1 and TRP2 [60]. Wang *et al.* [61] have reported that two phlegmacin type anthracenone dimer glycosides, auriculataosides A and B isolated from methanol extract of *Cassia auriculata* act as anti melanogenic agents. Auriculataosides A and B inhibited melanin synthesis by reducing tyrosinase, TRP1, TRP2, MITF protein expression.

5.3. Inhibition of Transfer of Melanosomes to Keratinocytes

There are various processes on which skin pigmentation regulation depends. The main factor that plays an essential role in cutaneous pigmentation is the transfer of melanosome to keratinocytes. So, in order to prevent hyperpigmentation, several treatment modes have been developed to inhibit melanosome transfer to keratinocytes.

Niacinamide which is a derivative of vitamin B3 is found in various foods such as milk, meat, vegetables, eggs, *etc.* In cocultures of melanocytes and keratinocytes, Greatens *et al.* [62] have showed that niacinamide inhibits transfer of melanosomes to keratinocytes. Through human clinical trial, they have concluded that niacinamide was able to reduce hyperpigmented macules. Methylophiopoganone B and Centaureidin (5,7,3'-trihydroxy-3,6,-'-trimethoxyflavone) isolated from two different plants Ophiopogon japonicas and Achillea millefolium respectively, were also found to inhibit melanosome transfer to keratinocytes [63, 64]. Ginsenosides, the major ingredients of ginseng affect pigment regulation by reducing melanin secretion and tyrosinase expression [65]. But, Lee *et al* [66]. have recently reported that Ginsenoside F1 isolated from ginseng plant showed antimelanogenic effect by inhibiting melanin transfer from melanocytes to keratinocytes. The list of plants discussed above is systematically represented in Table **1** with their active components and modes of action.

Table 1. Scientifically validated plants with their bioactive components having potential of skin whitening.

Plant	Active Component	Mode of Action	References
Cuminum cyminum	Cuminaldehyde	Inhibits oxidation of L-DOPA by tyrosinase	[21]
Galla rhois	1,2,3,4,6-PentaO galloyl-d-glucose (PGG)	Inhibits expression of MITF	[34]

(Table 1) cont.....

Plant	Active Component	Mode of Action	References
African medicinal plants (*Mondia whitei, Rhus vulgaris Meikle, Sclerocarya caffra*)	2-hydroxy-4-methoxybenzaldehyde	Inhibits oxidation of L-DOPA by tyrosinase	[22]
Cinnamomum cassia	Transcinnamaldehyde	Inhibits oxidation of L-tyrosine by tyrosinase	[23]
Pulsatilla cernua	3,4-dihydroxycinnamic acid, 4-hydroxy-3-methoxycinnamic acid	Inhibits oxidation of L-DOPA by tyrosinase	[24]
Panax ginseng	p-coumaric acid, Vanillic acid Ginsenoside F1	Inhibits oxidation of L-tyrosine by tyrosinase. Inhibits expression of MITF Reduces melanosome transfer to keratinocytes	[30] [56] [42]
Camellia sinensis	Epicatechin gallate, gallocatechin gallate, epigallocatechin gallate	Flavon-3-ol skeleton with galloyl moiety inhibits oxidation of L-DOPA by tyrosinase	[37]
Carthamus tinctorius	N-feruloyserotonin, N-(p-coumaroyl) serotonin acacetin	Inhibits expression of TYR, TRP-1, TRP-2	[45]
Ophiopogon japonicas	Methylphiopoganone B	Reduces melanosome transfer to keratinocytes	[63]
Achillea millefolium	Centaureidin	Reduces melanosome transfer to keratinocytes	[64]
Polygonum hydropiper	Taxifolin	Inhibits tyrosinase activity	[38]
Myristica fragrans	Macelignan	Inhibits expression of TYR, TRP-1, TRP-2	[46]
Astragalus membranaceus	Calycosin	Inhibits expression of TYR	[47]
Rosa canica	Quercetin	Inhibits expression of TYR, TRP-1, TRP-2	[48]
Kaempferia pandulata	Panduratin A	Inhibits expression of TYR, TRP-1, TRP-2	[49]
Polygonum cuspidatum	Piceid	Reduces expression of tyrosinase	[50]
Rehmania glutinosa	Acteoside	Reduces level of TYR, TRP-1, TRP-2, MITF	[52]
Ishige foliacae	Octaphlorethol A	Decreases TYR, TRP-1, TRP-2, MITF expression	[53]

(Table 1) cont.....

Plant	Active Component	Mode of Action	References
Caesalpinia sappan	Brazeilin	Inhibits oxidation of L-DOPA by tyrosinase	[39]
Pterocarpus santalinus	Santalin	Inhibits oxidation of L-DOPA by tyrosinase	[40]
Apis mellifera	10-hydroxy-2-decenoic acid (10-HDA)	Reduces expression of TYR, TRP-1, TRP-2	[57]
Sageretia thea	Methyl linoleate, methyl linolenate	Reduces expression of TYR, TRP-1, TRP-2, MITF	[58]
Glycyrrhiza uralensis	Dehyroglyasperin C	Reduces expression of TYR, TRP-1, TRP-2, MITF	[59]
Sophora flavescens	Kushenol-A, 8-prenylkaempferol	Inhibits oxidation of L-DOPA by tyrosinase	[41]
Sargassum serratifolium	Sargaquinoic acid	Reduces expression of TYR, TRP-1, TRP-2, MITF	[60]
Cassia auriculata	Auriculataosides A and B	Reduces expression of TYR, TRP-1, TRP-2, MITF	[61]
Lepechinia meyenii	Coumaric acid, caffeic acid, rosmarinic acid	Inhibits tyrosinase activity	[44]

6. SKIN WHITENING INGREDIENTS EXTRACTED FROM NATURAL SOURCES OTHER THAN PLANTS

Although plants are the rich treasure of medicines, but the use of microorganisms in medical sciences has also achieved enumerable success. In addition to the extraction of antibiotics from microorganisms, there are extraction of other compounds too as they can also possess certain compounds with other activities of pharmaceutically important. So, besides plants, some compounds from fungal sources have also been identified and reported for their antimelanogenic activity [67].

Yeast, *Pityrosporum ovale* was found to produced azelaic acid (1,7-heptanedi carboxylic acid), which is a naturally occurring straight chain, saturated dicarboxylic acid. Azelaic acid showed cytotoxic effect on malignant melanocytes of primary cutaneous melanoma without affecting the normal melanocytes [67]. Many species of *Aspergillus niger* and *Penicillium* are able to produce a fungal metabolite, kojic acid which is chemically a 5-hydroxy2-(hydroxymethyl) gamma-pyrone. Kojic acid is a good chelator of transition metal ions [68] and a good scavenger of free radicals and hence used to treat hyperpigmentation [69]. Kojic acid is one of the most widely used chemical analogues in skin whitening formulations [70]. Madhosingh and Sundberg [71] have isolated and purified two compounds from the mushroom *Agaricus hortensis*, which was characterized as tyrosinase inhibitors. Inhibitor 1a showed competitive inhibition, whereas 1b showed noncompetitive inhibition with tyrosinase.

Copper-metallothionein extracted from *Neurospora crassa* was reported as a metal donor for apotyrosinase. Metallothioneins of yeast are ubiquitous cytosolic proteins, characterized by selective binding of the huge amount of heavy metals and a high content of cysteine [72]. Metallothionein isolated from fungus *Aspergillus niger* was also reported to have tyrosinase inhibiting capability as it has a strong affinity to chelate copper at the active site of mushroom tyrosinase [73]. Studies showed that several other fungi such as *Phellinus linteus* [74], *Dictyophora indusiata* [75], *Daedalea dickinsii* [76] *Trichoderma viridae* [77], *Aspergillus niger* [78], *Paecylomyces gunnii* [79], *Neolentinus lepideus* [80] have been reported to produce tyrosinase inhibitory compounds. Additionally, tyrosinase inhibitors have been isolated from marine derived fungus also. Li *et al.* [81] have isolated myrothenones A and b and cyclopentone derivatives with tyrosinase inhibitory activity from the marine fungus *Myrothecium* sp. Similarly, Wu *et al.* [82] have isolated two novel tyrosinase inhibitory sesquiterpenes induced by $CuCl_2$ from marine derived fungus *Pestalotiopsi*s sp.

In addition to fungal derived tyrosinase inhibitors, there are several reports on inhibition of tyrosinase by different bacterial species and their metabolites. Streptomyces sp such as *S. hiroshimensis* isolated from soil [83], actinobacteria *Streptomyces roseolilacinus* [84] and *Streptomyces swartbergensis* [85] are the source of tyrosinase inhibitors. Some tyrosinase inhibitors are reported from a toxic strain of the Cyanobacterium, *Oscillatoria agardhii* [86] and a gram negative marine bacterium, *Thalassotalea* sp [87]. Interestingly, the probiotics such as *Lactobacillus* sp that are used in the fermentation process have also found to produce tyrosinase inhibitors. It has been confirmed from the studies that the physiological activities of fermented extracts were significantly higher than that of unfermented extracts, but their cytotoxicity was lower in fermented extracts [88]. Recently, Ji *et al.* [89] have extracted tyrosinase inhibitors from four different lactic acid bacteria (LAB) strains which were isolated from dairy cow faeces. The other tyrosinase inhibitors from microorganisms have been summarized in an updated review by Fernandes *et al.* [90].

CONCLUSION

As enzyme tyrosinase has a vital role in the process of melanogenesis, its inhibitors have been considered by the researchers in order to treat hyperpigmentation problems. Due to the side effects associated with synthetic and semi-synthetic compounds, natural sources, including plants and micrororganisms have been studied for their wonderful potential as anti tyrosinase agents. Nevertheless, the majority of the compounds have been isolated from plants, but microorganisms are also considered as a novel source of tyrosinase inhibitors. Most of the tyrosinase inhibitors isolated from natural sources are chemically phenolic compounds. Despite many compounds isolated from natural sources are successfully identified as tyrosinase inhibitors, there are several medicinal plants and many microorganisms which yet have to be studied for the antimelanogenic activities of their compounds. The field is wide open and seems to be highly promising provided proper scientific validation to be carried out before their claim as potent therapeutic agents.

REFERENCES

[1]   Ali, S.A.; Naaz, I. Current challenges in understanding the story of skin pigmentation: Bridging the morpho-anatomical and functional aspects of mammalian melanocytes. In: *Muscle Cell and Tissue*; Kunihiro, Sakuma, Ed.; InTech Open House: Europe, USA, **2015**; pp. 262-285.

[2]   Maddodi, N.; Jayanthy, A.; Setaluri, V. Shining light on skin pigmentation: the darker and the brighter side of effects of UV radiation. *Photochem. Photobiol.,* **2012**, *88*(5), 1075-1082.
[http://dx.doi.org/10.1111/j.1751-1097.2012.01138.x] [PMID: 22404235]

[3]   Vera Cruz, G. The impact of face skin tone on perceived facial attractiveness: A study realized with an innovative methodology. *J. Soc. Psychol.,* **2018**, *158*(5), 580-590.
[http://dx.doi.org/10.1080/00224545.2017.1419161] [PMID: 29257930]

[4]   Briganti, S.; Camera, E.; Picardo, M. Chemical and instrumental approaches to treat hyperpigmentation. *Pigment Cell Res.,* **2003**, *16*(2), 101-110.
[http://dx.doi.org/10.1034/j.1600-0749.2003.00029.x] [PMID: 12622786]

[5]   Tadokoro, T.; Bonté, F.; Archambault, J.C.; Cauchard, J.H.; Neveu, M.; Ozawa, K.; Noguchi, F.; Ikeda, A.; Nagamatsu, M.; Shinn, S. Whitening efficacy of plant extracts including orchid extracts on Japanese female skin with melasma and lentigo senilis. *J. Dermatol.,* **2010**, *37*(6), 522-530.
[http://dx.doi.org/10.1111/j.1346-8138.2010.00897.x] [PMID: 20536665]

[6]   Gunia-Krzyżak, A.; Popiol, J.; Marona, H. Melanogenesis Inhibitors: Strategies for Searching for and Evaluation of Active Compounds. *Curr. Med. Chem.,* **2016**, *23*(31), 3548-3574.
[http://dx.doi.org/10.2174/0929867323666160627094938] [PMID: 27356545]

[7]   Kanlayavattanakul, M.; Lourith, N. Skin hyperpigmentation treatment using herbs: A review of clinical evidences. *J. Cosmet. Laser Ther.,* **2018**, *20*(2), 123-131.
[http://dx.doi.org/10.1080/14764172.2017.1368666] [PMID: 28853960]

[8]   Ali, S.A. Recent advances in treatment of skin disorders using herbal products. *J. Skin,* **2017**, *1*(1), 6-7.

[9]   Kanlayavattanakul, M.; Lourith, N. Plants and Natural Products for the Treatment of Skin Hyperpigmentation - A Review. *Planta Med.,* **2018**, *84*(14), 988-1006.
[http://dx.doi.org/10.1055/a-0583-0410] [PMID: 29506294]

[10]   Elmets, C.A.; Anderson, C.Y. Sunscreens and photocarcinogenesis: an objective assessment.

Photochem. Photobiol., **1996**, *63*(4), 435-440.
[http://dx.doi.org/10.1111/j.1751-1097.1996.tb03065.x] [PMID: 8934759]

[11]   An, S.M.; Koh, J.S.; Boo, Y.C. p-coumaric acid not only inhibits human tyrosinase activity *in vitro* but also melanogenesis in cells exposed to UVB. *Phytother. Res.,* **2010**, *24*(8), 1175-1180.
[http://dx.doi.org/10.1002/ptr.3095] [PMID: 20077437]

[12]   Ali, S.A.; Choudhary, R.K.; Naaz, I.; Ali, A.S. Understanding the Challenges of Melanogenesis: Key Role of Bioactive Compounds in the Treatment of Hyperpigmentory Disorders. *J. Pigment. Disord.,* **2015**, *2*(11), 1-9.

[13]   Vashi, N.A.; Kundu, R.V. Facial hyperpigmentation: causes and treatment. *Br. J. Dermatol.,* **2013**, *169*(3) Suppl. 3, 41-56.
[http://dx.doi.org/10.1111/bjd.12536] [PMID: 24098900]

[14]   Pérez-Bernal, A.; Muñoz-Pérez, M.A.; Camacho, F. Management of facial hyperpigmentation. *Am. J. Clin. Dermatol.,* **2000**, *1*(5), 261-268.
[http://dx.doi.org/10.2165/00128071-200001050-00001] [PMID: 11702317]

[15]   Rigopoulos, D.; Gregoriou, S.; Katsambas, A. Hyperpigmentation and melasma. *J. Cosmet. Dermatol.,* **2007**, *6*(3), 195-202.
[http://dx.doi.org/10.1111/j.1473-2165.2007.00321.x] [PMID: 17760699]

[16]   Shamsaldeen, O.; Peterson, J.D.; Goldman, M.P. The adverse events of deep fractional CO(2): a retrospective study of 490 treatments in 374 patients. *Lasers Surg. Med.,* **2011**, *43*(6), 453-456.
[http://dx.doi.org/10.1002/lsm.21079] [PMID: 21761414]

[17]   Costa, I.M.C.; Damasceno, P.S.; Costa, M.C.; Gomes, K.G.P. Review in peeling complications. *J. Cosmet. Dermatol.,* **2017**, *16*(3), 319-326.
[http://dx.doi.org/10.1111/jocd.12329] [PMID: 28349655]

[18]   Magalhães, G.M.; Rodrigues, D.F.; Oliveira, E.R.; Ferreira, F.A.A. Tretinoin peeling: when a reaction is greater than expected. *An. Bras. Dermatol.,* **2017**, *92*(2), 291-292.
[http://dx.doi.org/10.1590/abd1806-4841.20176728] [PMID: 28538908]

[19]   Libon, F.; Courtois, J.; Le Goff, C.; Lukas, P.; Fabregat-Cabello, N.; Seidel, L.; Cavalier, E.; Nikkels, A.F. Sunscreens block cutaneous vitamin D production with only a minimal effect on circulating 25-hydroxyvitamin D. *Arch. Osteoporos.,* **2017**, *12*(1), 66.
[http://dx.doi.org/10.1007/s11657-017-0361-0] [PMID: 28718005]

[20]   Gillbro, J.M.; Olsson, M.J. The melanogenesis and mechanisms of skin-lightening agents--existing and new approaches. *Int. J. Cosmet. Sci.,* **2011**, *33*(3), 210-221.
[http://dx.doi.org/10.1111/j.1468-2494.2010.00616.x] [PMID: 21265866]

[21]   Kubo, I.; Kinst-Hori, I. Tyrosinase inhibitors from cumin. *J. Agric. Food Chem.,* **1988**, *46*, 5338-5341.
[http://dx.doi.org/10.1021/jf980226+]

[22]   Kubo, I.; Kinst-Hori, I. 2-Hydroxy-4-methoxybenzaldehyde: a potent tyrosinase inhibitor from African medicinal plants. *Planta Med.,* **1999**, *65*(1), 19-22.
[http://dx.doi.org/10.1055/s-1999-13955] [PMID: 10083839]

[23]   Lee, S.E.; Kim, M.O.; Lee, S.G.; Ahn, Y.J.; Lee, H.S. Inhibitory effects of *Cinnamomum cassia* bark-derived materials on mushroom tyrosinase. *Food Sci. Biotechnol.,* **2000**, *9*, 330-333.

[24]   Lee, H.S. Tyrosinase inhibitors of *Pulsatilla cernua* root-derived materials. *J. Agric. Food Chem.,* **2002**, *50*(6), 1400-1403.
[http://dx.doi.org/10.1021/jf011230f] [PMID: 11879010]

[25]   Ha, T.J.; Tamura, S.; Kubo, I. Effects of mushroom tyrosinase on anisaldehyde. *J. Agric. Food Chem.,* **2005**, *53*(18), 7024-7028.
[http://dx.doi.org/10.1021/jf047943q] [PMID: 16131106]

[26]   Kubo, I.; Yokokawa, Y. Two tyrosinase inhibiting flavonol glycosides from *Buddleia coriacea.*

Phytochemistry, **1992**, *31*, 1075-1077.
[http://dx.doi.org/10.1016/0031-9422(92)80084-R]

[27]   Kubo, I.; Kinst-Hori, I.; Yokokawa, Y. Tyrosinase inhibitors from *Anacardium occidentale* fruits. *J. Nat. Prod.,* **1994**, *57*(4), 545-551.
[http://dx.doi.org/10.1021/np50106a021] [PMID: 8021657]

[28]   Kubo, I.; Kinst-Hori, I. Flavonols from saffron flower: tyrosinase inhibitory activity and inhibition mechanism. *J. Agric. Food Chem.,* **1999**, *47*(10), 4121-4125.
[http://dx.doi.org/10.1021/jf990201q] [PMID: 10552777]

[29]   Chen, Q.X.; Kubo, I. Kinetics of mushroom tyrosinase inhibition by quercetin. *J. Agric. Food Chem.,* **2002**, *50*(14), 4108-4112.
[http://dx.doi.org/10.1021/jf011378z] [PMID: 12083892]

[30]   Lim, J.Y.; Ishiguro, K.; Kubo, I. Tyrosinase inhibitory p-coumaric acid from ginseng leaves. *Phytother. Res.,* **1999**, *13*(5), 371-375.
[http://dx.doi.org/10.1002/(SICI)1099-1573(199908/09)13:5<371::AID-PTR453>3.0.CO;2-L] [PMID: 10441774]

[31]   Boo, Y.C. *p*-Coumaric Acid as An Active Ingredient in Cosmetics: A Review Focusing on its Antimelanogenic Effects. *Antioxidants,* **2019**, *8*(8), E275.
[http://dx.doi.org/10.3390/antiox8080275] [PMID: 31382682]

[32]   Shin, N.H.; Ryu, S.Y.; Choi, E.J.; Kang, S.H.; Chang, I.M.; Min, K.R.; Kim, Y. Oxyresveratrol as the potent inhibitor on dopa oxidase activity of mushroom tyrosinase. *Biochem. Biophys. Res. Commun.,* **1998**, *243*(3), 801-803.
[http://dx.doi.org/10.1006/bbrc.1998.8169] [PMID: 9500997]

[33]   Badria, F.A.; elGayyar, M.A. A new type of tyrosinase inhibitors from natural products as potential treatments for hyperpigmentation. *Boll. Chim. Farm.,* **2001**, *140*(4), 267-271.
[PMID: 11570225]

[34]   Kim, J.H.; Sapers, G.M.; Choi, S.W. Identification of tyrosinase inhibitor from Galla rhois. *Food Sci. Biotechnol.,* **1998**, *7*, 56-59.

[35]   Menon, S.; Fleck, R.W.; Yong, G.; Strothkamp, K.G. Benzoic acid inhibition of the alpha, β, and γ isozymes of Agaricus bisporus tyrosinase. *Arch. Biochem. Biophys.,* **1990**, *280*(1), 27-32.
[http://dx.doi.org/10.1016/0003-9861(90)90513-X] [PMID: 2112900]

[36]   Kermasha, S.; Goetghebeur, M.; Monfette, A.; Metchet, M.; Rovelt, M. Inhibitory effects of cysteine and aromatic acids on tyrosinase activity. *Phytochemistry,* **1993**, *34*, 349-353.
[http://dx.doi.org/10.1016/0031-9422(93)80007-F]

[37]   No, J.K.; Soung, D.Y.; Kim, Y.J.; Shim, K.H.; Jun, Y.S.; Rhee, S.H.; Yokozawa, T.; Chung, H.Y. Inhibition of tyrosinase by green tea components. *Life Sci.,* **1999**, *65*(21), PL241-PL246.
[http://dx.doi.org/10.1016/S0024-3205(99)00492-0] [PMID: 10576599]

[38]   Miyazawa, M.; Tamura, N. Inhibitory compound of tyrosinase activity from the sprout of *Polygonum hydropiper* L. (Benitade). *Biol. Pharm. Bull.,* **2007**, *30*(3), 595-597.
[http://dx.doi.org/10.1248/bpb.30.595] [PMID: 17329865]

[39]   Hridya, H.; Amrita, A.; Sankari, M.; George Priya Doss, C.; Gopalakrishnan, M.; Gopalakrishnan, C.; Siva, R. Inhibitory effect of brazilein on tyrosinase and melanin synthesis: Kinetics and *in silico* approach. *Int. J. Biol. Macromol.,* **2015**, *81*, 228-234.
[http://dx.doi.org/10.1016/j.ijbiomac.2015.07.064] [PMID: 26254246]

[40]   Hridya, H.; Amrita, A.; Mohan, S.; Gopalakrishnan, M.; Dakshinamurthy, T.K.; Doss, G.P.; Siva, R. Functionality study of santalin as tyrosinase inhibitor: A potential depigmentation agent. *Int. J. Biol. Macromol.,* **2016**, *86*, 383-389.
[http://dx.doi.org/10.1016/j.ijbiomac.2016.01.098] [PMID: 26828288]

[41]   Kim, J.H.; Cho, I.S.; So, Y.K.; Kim, H.H.; Kim, Y.H. Kushenol A and 8-prenylkaempferol, tyrosinase

inhibitors, derived from *Sophora flavescens. J. Enzyme Inhib. Med. Chem.,* **2018**, *33*(1), 1048-1054.
[http://dx.doi.org/10.1080/14756366.2018.1477776] [PMID: 29873272]

[42]	Lee, H.J.; Sim, M.O.; Woo, K.W.; Jeong, D.E.; Jung, H.K.; An, B.; Cho, H.W. Antioxidant and Antimelanogenic Activities of Compounds Isolated from the Aerial Parts of *Achillea alpina* L. *Chem. Biodivers.,* **2019**, *16*(7), e1900033.
[http://dx.doi.org/10.1002/cbdv.201900033] [PMID: 30977279]

[43]	Tang, M.; Hou, F.; Wu, Y.; Liu, Y.; Ouyang, J. Purification, characterization and tyrosinase inhibition activity of polysaccharides from chestnut (Castanea mollissima Bl.) kernel. *Int. J. Biol. Macromol.,* **2019**, *131*, 309-314.
[http://dx.doi.org/10.1016/j.ijbiomac.2019.03.065] [PMID: 30872058]

[44]	Crespo, M.I.; Chabán, M.F.; Lanza, P.A.; Joray, M.B.; Palacios, S.M.; Vera, D.M.A.; Carpinella, M.C. Inhibitory effects of compounds isolated from *Lepechinia meyenii* on tyrosinase. *Food Chem. Toxicol.,* **2019**, *125*(125), 383-391.
[http://dx.doi.org/10.1016/j.fct.2019.01.019] [PMID: 30684603]

[45]	Roh, J.S.; Han, J.Y.; Kim, J.H.; Hwang, J.K. Inhibitory effects of active compounds isolated from safflower (*Carthamus tinctorius* L.) seeds for melanogenesis. *Biol. Pharm. Bull.,* **2004**, *27*(12), 1976-1978.
[http://dx.doi.org/10.1248/bpb.27.1976] [PMID: 15577216]

[46]	Cho, Y.; Kim, K.H.; Shim, J.S.; Hwang, J.K. Inhibitory effects of macelignan isolated from *Myristica fragrans* HOUTT. on melanin biosynthesis. *Biol. Pharm. Bull.,* **2008**, *31*(5), 986-989.
[http://dx.doi.org/10.1248/bpb.31.986] [PMID: 18451531]

[47]	Kim, J.H.; Kim, M.R.; Lee, E.S.; Lee, C.H. Inhibitory effects of calycosin isolated from the root of *Astragalus membranaceus* on melanin biosynthesis. *Biol. Pharm. Bull.,* **2009**, *32*(2), 264-268.
[http://dx.doi.org/10.1248/bpb.32.264] [PMID: 19182387]

[48]	Fujii, T.; Saito, M. Inhibitory effect of quercetin isolated from rose hip (*Rosa canina* L.) against melanogenesis by mouse melanoma cells. *Biosci. Biotechnol. Biochem.,* **2009**, *73*(9), 1989-1993.
[http://dx.doi.org/10.1271/bbb.90181] [PMID: 19734679]

[49]	Lee, C.W.; Kim, H.S.; Kim, H.K.; Kim, J.W.; Yoon, J.H.; Cho, Y.; Hwang, J.K. Inhibitory effect of panduratin A isolated from *Kaempferia panduarata* Roxb. on melanin biosynthesis. *Phytother. Res.,* **2010**, *24*(11), 1600-1604.
[http://dx.doi.org/10.1002/ptr.3163] [PMID: 21031615]

[50]	Jeong, E.T.; Jin, M.H.; Kim, M.S.; Chang, Y.H.; Park, S.G. Inhibition of melanogenesis by piceid isolated from *Polygonum cuspidatum. Arch. Pharm. Res.,* **2010**, *33*(9), 1331-1338.
[http://dx.doi.org/10.1007/s12272-010-0906-x] [PMID: 20945131]

[51]	Lee, J.H.; Jang, J.Y.; Park, C.; Kim, B.W.; Choi, Y.H.; Choi, B.T. Curcumin suppresses alpha-melanocyte stimulating hormone-stimulated melanogenesis in B16F10 cells. *Int. J. Mol. Med.,* **2010**, *26*(1), 101-106.
[PMID: 20514428]

[52]	Son, Y.O.; Lee, S.A.; Kim, S.S.; Jang, Y.S.; Chun, J.C.; Lee, J.C. Acteoside inhibits melanogenesis in B16F10 cells through ERK activation and tyrosinase down-regulation. *J. Pharm. Pharmacol.,* **2011**, *63*(10), 1309-1319.
[http://dx.doi.org/10.1111/j.2042-7158.2011.01335.x] [PMID: 21899547]

[53]	Kim, K.N.; Yang, H.M.; Kang, S.M.; Kim, D.; Ahn, G.; Jeon, Y.J. Octaphlorethol A isolated from *Ishige foliacea* inhibits α-MSH-stimulated induced melanogenesis *via* ERK pathway in B16F10 melanoma cells. *Food Chem. Toxicol.,* **2013**, *59*, 521-526.
[http://dx.doi.org/10.1016/j.fct.2013.06.031] [PMID: 23810793]

[54]	Nishina, A.; Ebina, K.; Ukiya, M.; Fukatsu, M.; Koketsu, M.; Ninomiya, M.; Sato, D.; Kimura, H. Dioscin Derived from Solanum melongena L. "Usukawamarunasu" Attenuates α-MSH-Induced Melanogenesis in B16 Murine Melanoma Cells *via* Downregulation of Phospho-CREB and MITF. *J.*

Food Sci., **2015**, *80*(10), H2354-H2359.
[http://dx.doi.org/10.1111/1750-3841.13068] [PMID: 26352003]

[55] Lee, D.Y.; Lee, J.; Jeong, Y.T.; Byun, G.H.; Kim, J.H. Melanogenesis inhibition activity of floralginsenoside A from *Panax ginseng* berry. *J. Ginseng Res.,* **2017**, *41*(4), 602-607.
[http://dx.doi.org/10.1016/j.jgr.2017.03.005] [PMID: 29021710]

[56] Liu, J.; Xu, X.; Jiang, R.; Sun, L.; Zhao, D. Vanillic acid in *Panax ginseng* root extract inhibits melanogenesis in B16F10 cells *via* inhibition of the NO/PKG signaling pathway. *Biosci. Biotechnol. Biochem.,* **2019**, *83*(7), 1205-1215.
[http://dx.doi.org/10.1080/09168451.2019.1606694] [PMID: 30999826]

[57] Peng, C.C.; Sun, H.T.; Lin, I.P.; Kuo, P.C.; Li, J.C. The functional property of royal jelly 10-hydrox--2-decenoic acid as a melanogenesis inhibitor. *BMC Complement. Altern. Med.,* **2017**, *17*(1), 392.
[http://dx.doi.org/10.1186/s12906-017-1888-8] [PMID: 28793915]

[58] Ko, G.A.; Shrestha, S.; Kim Cho, S. *Sageretia thea* fruit extracts rich in methyl linoleate and methyl linolenate downregulate melanogenesis *via* the Akt/GSK3β signaling pathway. *Nutr. Res. Pract.,* **2018**, *12*(1), 3-12.
[http://dx.doi.org/10.4162/nrp.2018.12.1.3] [PMID: 29399291]

[59] Lim, J.W.; Ha, J.H.; Jeong, Y.J.; Park, S.N. Anti-melanogenesis effect of dehydroglyasperin C through the downregulation of MITF *via* the reduction of intracellular cAMP and acceleration of ERK activation in B16F1 melanoma cells. *Pharmacol. Rep.,* **2018**, *70*(5), 930-935.
[http://dx.doi.org/10.1016/j.pharep.2018.02.024]

[60] Azam, M.S.; Kwon, M.; Choi, J.; Kim, H.R. Sargaquinoic acid ameliorates hyperpigmentation through cAMP and ERK-mediated downregulation of MITF in α-MSH-stimulated B16F10 cells. *Biomed. Pharmacother.,* **2018**, *104*, 582-589.
[http://dx.doi.org/10.1016/j.biopha.2018.05.083] [PMID: 29803170]

[61] Wang, W.; Zhang, Y.; Nakashima, S.; Nakamura, S.; Wang, T.; Yoshikawa, M.; Matsuda, H. Inhibition of melanin production by anthracenone dimer glycosides isolated from *Cassia auriculata* seeds. *J. Nat. Med.,* **2019**, *73*(3), 439-449.
[http://dx.doi.org/10.1007/s11418-018-01276-2] [PMID: 30847755]

[62] Greatens, A.; Hakozaki, T.; Koshoffer, A.; Epstein, H.; Schwemberger, S.; Babcock, G.; Bissett, D.; Takiwaki, H.; Arase, S.; Wickett, R.R.; Boissy, R.E. Effective inhibition of melanosome transfer to keratinocytes by lectins and niacinamide is reversible. *Exp. Dermatol.,* **2005**, *14*(7), 498-508.
[http://dx.doi.org/10.1111/j.0906-6705.2005.00309.x] [PMID: 15946237]

[63] Ito, Y.; Kanamaru, A.; Tada, A. Effects of methylophiopogonanone B on melanosome transfer and dendrite retraction. *J. Dermatol. Sci.,* **2006**, *42*(1), 68-70.
[http://dx.doi.org/10.1016/j.jdermsci.2005.12.015] [PMID: 16472989]

[64] Ito, Y.; Kanamaru, A.; Tada, A. Centaureidin promotes dendrite retraction of melanocytes by activating Rho. *Biochim. Biophys. Acta,* **2006**, *1760*(3), 487-494.
[http://dx.doi.org/10.1016/j.bbagen.2006.01.003] [PMID: 16476521]

[65] Kim, J.H.; Baek, E.J.; Lee, E.J.; Yeom, M.H.; Park, J.S.; Lee, K.W.; Kang, N.J. Ginsenoside F1 attenuates hyperpigmentation in B16F10 melanoma cells by inducing dendrite retraction and activating Rho signalling. *Exp. Dermatol.,* **2015**, *24*(2), 150-152.
[http://dx.doi.org/10.1111/exd.12586] [PMID: 25381719]

[66] Lee, C.S.; Nam, G.; Bae, I.H.; Park, J. Whitening efficacy of ginsenoside F1 through inhibition of melanin transfer in cocultured human melanocytes-keratinocytes and three-dimensional human skin equivalent. *J. Ginseng Res.,* **2019**, *43*(2), 300-304.
[http://dx.doi.org/10.1016/j.jgr.2017.12.005] [PMID: 30962737]

[67] Schallreuter, K.U.; Wood, J.W. A possible mechanism of action for azelaic acid in the human epidermis. *Arch. Dermatol. Res.,* **1990**, *282*(3), 168-171.
[http://dx.doi.org/10.1007/BF00372617] [PMID: 2114832]

[68] Parrish, F.W.; Wiley, B.J.; Simmons, E.G.; Long, L., Jr Production of aflatoxins and kojic acid by species of aspergillus and penicillium. *Appl. Microbiol.,* **1966**, *14*(1), 139.
[http://dx.doi.org/10.1128/AM.14.1.139-.1966] [PMID: 5914491]

[69] Wiley, J.W.; Tyson, G.N.; Steller, J.S. The configuration of complex kojates formed with some transition elements as determined by magnetic susceptibility measurements. *J. Am. Chem. Soc.,* **1942**, *64*, 963-964.
[http://dx.doi.org/10.1021/ja01256a062]

[70] Niwa, Y.; Akamatsu, H. Kojic acid scavenges free radicals while potentiating leukocyte functions including free radical generation. *Inflammation,* **1991**, *15*(4), 303-315.
[http://dx.doi.org/10.1007/BF00917315] [PMID: 1769733]

[71] Madhosingh, C.; Sundberg, L. Purification and properties of tyrosinase inhibitor from mushroom. *FEBS Lett.,* **1974**, *49*(2), 156-158.
[http://dx.doi.org/10.1016/0014-5793(74)80500-4] [PMID: 4216515]

[72] Lerch, K. Copper monooxygenases: Tyrosinase and dopamine β -monooxygenase. In: *Metal Ions in Biological Systems*; Sigel, H., Ed.; Dekker: New York, **1981**; pp. 143-186.

[73] Goetghebeur, M.; Kermasha, S. Inhibition of polyphenol oxidase by copper-metallothionein from *Aspergillus niger. Phytochemistry,* **1996**, *42*(4), 935-940.
[http://dx.doi.org/10.1016/0031-9422(96)86993-7] [PMID: 8688193]

[74] Kang, H.S.; Choi, J.H.; Cho, W.K.; Park, J.C.; Choi, J.S. A sphingolipid and tyrosinase inhibitors from the fruiting body of *Phellinus linteus. Arch. Pharm. Res.,* **2004**, *27*(7), 742-750.
[http://dx.doi.org/10.1007/BF02980143] [PMID: 15357002]

[75] Sharma, V.K.; Choi, J.; Sharma, N.; Choi, M.; Seo, S.Y. *In vitro* anti-tyrosinase activity of 5-(hydroxymethyl)-2-furfural isolated from *Dictyophora indusiata. Phytother. Res.,* **2004**, *18*(10), 841-844.
[http://dx.doi.org/10.1002/ptr.1428] [PMID: 15551389]

[76] Morimura, K.; Yamazaki, C.; Hattori, Y.; Makabe, H.; Kamo, T.; Hirota, M. A tyrosinase inhibitor, Daedalin A, from mycelial culture of *Daedalea dickinsii. Biosci. Biotechnol. Biochem.,* **2007**, *71*(11), 2837-2840.
[http://dx.doi.org/10.1271/bbb.70266] [PMID: 17986791]

[77] Tsuchiya, T.; Yamada, K.; Minoura, K.; Miyamoto, K.; Usami, Y.; Kobayashi, T.; Hamada-Sato, N.; Imada, C.; Tsujibo, H. Purification and determination of the chemical structure of the tyrosinase inhibitor produced by *Trichoderma viride* strain H1-7 from a marine environment. *Biol. Pharm. Bull.,* **2008**, *31*(8), 1618-1620.
[http://dx.doi.org/10.1248/bpb.31.1618] [PMID: 18670100]

[78] Vasantha, K.Y.; Murugesh, C.S.; Sattur, A.P. A tyrosinase inhibitor from *Aspergillus niger. J. Food Sci. Technol.,* **2014**, *51*(10), 2877-2880.
[http://dx.doi.org/10.1007/s13197-014-1395-6] [PMID: 25328242]

[79] Lu, R.; Liu, X.; Gao, S.; Zhang, W.; Peng, F.; Hu, F.; Huang, B.; Chen, L.; Bao, G.; Li, C.; Li, Z. New tyrosinase inhibitors from *Paecilomyces gunnii. J. Agric. Food Chem.,* **2014**, *62*(49), 11917-11923.
[http://dx.doi.org/10.1021/jf504128c] [PMID: 25384266]

[80] Ishihara, A.; Ide, Y.; Bito, T.; Ube, N.; Endo, N.; Sotome, K.; Maekawa, N.; Ueno, K.; Nakagiri, A. Novel tyrosinase inhibitors from liquid culture of *Neolentinus lepideus. Biosci. Biotechnol. Biochem.,* **2018**, *82*(1), 22-30.
[http://dx.doi.org/10.1080/09168451.2017.1415125] [PMID: 29297258]

[81] Li, X.; Kim, M.K.; Lee, U.; Kim, S.K.; Kang, J.S.; Choi, H.D.; Son, B.W. Myrothenones A and B, cyclopentenone derivatives with tyrosinase inhibitory activity from the marine-derived fungus *Myrothecium* sp. *Chem. Pharm. Bull. (Tokyo),* **2005**, *53*(4), 453-455.
[http://dx.doi.org/10.1248/cpb.53.453] [PMID: 15802853]

[82]   Wu, B.; Wu, X.; Sun, M.; Li, M. Two novel tyrosinase inhibitory sesquiterpenes induced by CuCl2 from a marine-derived fungus *Pestalotiopsis* sp. Z233. *Mar. Drugs,* **2013**, *11*(8), 2713-2721.
[http://dx.doi.org/10.3390/md11082713] [PMID: 23917067]

[83]   Chang, T.S.; Tseng, M.; Ding, H.Y.; Shou-Ku Tai, S. Isolation and characterization of Streptomyces hiroshimensis strain TI-C3 with anti-tyrosinase activity. *J. Cosmet. Sci.,* **2008**, *59*(1), 33-40.
[PMID: 18350233]

[84]   Nakashima, T.; Anzai, K.; Kuwahara, N.; Komaki, H.; Miyadoh, S.; Harayama, S.; Tianero, M.D.; Tanaka, J.; Kanamoto, A.; Ando, K. Physicochemical characters of a tyrosinase inhibitor produced by *Streptomyces roseolilacinus* NBRC 12815. *Biol. Pharm. Bull.,* **2009**, *32*(5), 832-836.
[http://dx.doi.org/10.1248/bpb.32.832] [PMID: 19420750]

[85]   le Roes-Hill, M.; Prins, A.; Meyers, P.R. *Streptomyces swartbergensis* sp. nov., a novel tyrosinase and antibiotic producing actinobacterium. *Antonie van Leeuwenhoek,* **2018**, *111*(4), 589-600.
[http://dx.doi.org/10.1007/s10482-017-0979-3] [PMID: 29110155]

[86]   Sano, T.; Kaya, K. Oscillapeptin G, a tyrosinase inhibitor from toxic Oscillatoria agardhii. *J. Nat. Prod.,* **1996**, *59*(1), 90-92.
[http://dx.doi.org/10.1021/np9600210] [PMID: 8984160]

[87]   Deering, R.W.; Chen, J.; Sun, J.; Ma, H.; Dubert, J.; Barja, J.L.; Seeram, N.P.; Wang, H.; Rowley, D.C. N-acyl dehydrotyrosines, tyrosinase inhibitors from the marine bacterium *Thalassotalea* sp. PP2-459. *J. Nat. Prod.,* **2016**, *79*(2), 447-450.
[http://dx.doi.org/10.1021/acs.jnatprod.5b00972] [PMID: 26824128]

[88]   Wang, G.H.; Chen, C.Y.; Tsai, T.H.; Chen, C.K.; Cheng, C.Y.; Huang, Y.H.; Hsieh, M.C.; Chung, Y.C. Evaluation of tyrosinase inhibitory and antioxidant activities of Angelica dahurica root extracts for four different probiotic bacteria fermentations. *J. Biosci. Bioeng.,* **2017**, *123*(6), 679-684.
[http://dx.doi.org/10.1016/j.jbiosc.2017.01.003] [PMID: 28254340]

[89]   Ji, K.; Cho, Y.S.; Kim, Y.T. Tyrosinase inhibitory and anti-oxidative effects of lactic acid bacteria isolated from dairy cow feces. *Probiotics Antimicrob. Proteins,* **2018**, *10*(1), 43-55.
[http://dx.doi.org/10.1007/s12602-017-9274-x] [PMID: 28478573]

[90]   Fernandes, M.S.; Kerkar, S. Microorganisms as a source of tyrosinase inhibitors: a review. *Ann. Microbiol.,* **2017**, *67*, 343-358.
[http://dx.doi.org/10.1007/s13213-017-1261-7]

CHAPTER 9

Role of Computational Tools to Evaluate Potent Tyrosinase Inhibitors used for the Treatment of Skin Hyperpigmentation

Abstract: Melanin pigment has a photo defensive role in human skin, but its redundant production and distribution lead to the problem of hyperpigmentation. Biosynthesis of melanin initiated from tyrosine oxidation through the key enzyme tyrosinase. In addition to human and animal, tyrosinase is broadly distributed in plants also and is responsible for browning of fruits and vegetables. Quest for the search of tyrosinase inhibitors is significant to enable the development of therapies for the prevention and treatment of hyperpigmentation and the undesirable browning of fruits and vegetables. Various synthetic and natural compounds have been tested for their inhibitory activity but the mechanism of inhibition is not known so far, and there is a continuous hunt for information concerning intermolecular interaction between inhibitors and tyrosinase. Thus, computer aided methods are consequently used to overwhelmed such issues. *In silico* methods such as molecular docking simulation, make it possible to understand the intermolecular interaction between inhibitors and tyrosinase, and hence, help identify new and potent tyrosinase inhibitors. The present chapter has pointed out the role of computational tools for the elucidation of tyrosinase inhibitors, highlighting the examples of certain compounds whose antityrosinase activities have been evaluated using molecular docking algorithms.

Keywords: Computer aided, Hyperpigmentation, Melanin, Molecular docking, Tyrosinase.

1. INTRODUCTION

Due to the presence of melanin, human skin acts as a barrier from different ionizing radiations like UV radiation. In addition, to provide protection from UV radiation, melanin also absorbs free radicals found in the cytoplasm of melanocytes. Melanin is produced inside the specialized organelles, melanosomes of melanocytes by a complex process of melanogenesis through a series of enzymatic and chemical reactions. Synthesis and distribution of melanin regulate the color of our skin [1]. But, the rise in production and accumulation of melanin in different parts of the skin leads to various aesthetic problems in the form of hyperpigmentation. The various forms of hyperpigmentation, including melasma,

Sharique A. Ali & Naima Parveen

senile, ephelides, freckles, lentigines, *etc.* have been observed due to excess melanin production in the skin [2, 3].

Tyrosinase, tyrosinase related protein-1 (TRP-1), and tyrosinase related protein-2 (TRP-2), *etc.* are the enzymes which are involved in melanogenesis pathway. But tyrosinase is known as the key enzyme of melanogenesis because it catalyzes the rate limiting reaction of melanogenesis [4]. Accordingly, to treat hyperpigmentation, different inhibitors of tyrosinase have been evaluated [5]. In addition to having a role in animal and human skin pigmentation, enzyme tyrosinase is widely distributed in plants also. In plants, its function is to control the quality of vegetables and fruits. Tyrosinase catalyze the phenolic compounds oxidation to the respective quinines, hence liable for early browning of fruits and vegetables which is not desired [6].

Different compounds have been tested for their tyrosinase inhibitory activity originated from both natural and synthetic sources. Some of them inhibit tyrosinase but their action mechanisms are not specific and there is little information on tyrosinase-inhibitors intermolecular interactions. More studies on tyrosinase and their inhibitors are required to well understand the inhibition mechanisms [7]. The use of computer aided methods like Quantitative structure activity relationship (QSAR) based virtual screening makes it possible to overcome such issues [8].

Computational studies have become more popular and complementary to experiments in wet laboratory in identifying the structure and function of complex biomolecules [9]. Molecular docking strategy is a frequently used tool in structure based drug design. It identifies the possible bindings of two molecules. Hence this can be used for the identification and development of specific and potent target inhibitors of tyrosinase [10, 11]. Therefore, in contrast to *in vitro* and *in vivo* studies, here in this chapter, we have focused our attention on the use of computational methods to elucidate novel and potent agents having tyrosinase inhibitory activity.

2. TYROSINASE: STRUCTURAL PROPERTIES AND ROLE IN MELANOGENESIS

An enzyme tyrosinase (EC 1.14.18.1) is a mono or diphenol oxidoreductase. It is a well-known copper containing enzyme of the oxidase superfamily, which is responsible for skin pigmentation as it involved in the synthesis of melanin pigment in vertebrates [12 - 14]. Tyrosinase is known to catalyse two major reactions of melanin synthesis. First reaction is the production of 3,4 dihydroxy phenylalanine (DOPA) which is a diphenol from tyrosine which is monophenol by hydroxylation reaction. In the second reaction, DOPA is converted into corresponding o-quinone or dopaquinone. o-quinone is very reactive and through a series of reactions, it can polymerize to form high molecular weight compounds in the form of black/brown pigment known as melanin [15, 16].

Tyrosinase is categorized as type III copper enzyme as it contains two coupled copper cations, each of which is coordinated by histidine imidazoles in their active sites, whose role is to derive dioxygen to initiate catalytic activity [17]. The pair of copper cations situated within the active site of tyrosinase interacts with atmospheric oxygen and start catalysing two types of reactions: (i) ortho-hydroxylation of monophenols and (ii) oxidation of o-diphenol to o-quinones [18, 19].

The first report of three dimensional structure of tyrosinase was given by Matoba *et al.* [20]. They have revealed the structure of *Streptomyces castaneoglobisporus* tyrosinase with PDB ID: 1WX2. A bacteria *Bacillus megaterium* was used to resolve the structure of its tyrosinase with PDB ID: 3NM8 [21]. Ismaya *et al.* [22] have solved the 3D structure of *Agaricus bisporus* (mushroom) tyrosinase with PDB ID: 2Y9W. They have observed that tyrosinase is a tetramer with two light and two heavy chains. It is evident from the above discussed three studies that 3D structure of tyrosinase is typically I-helical. A small parallel sheet structure was formed by the two u- strands at the N and C terminus of catalytic domain of tyrosinase. The four helix bundles formed the core of an enzyme, in which binuclear copper is present.

The first structure of plant tyrosinase was revealed by X-ray crystallography to a resolution of 1.8 A. Tyrosinase used for the structure elucidation was extracted by two phase extraction method from the leaves of a walnut plant (*Juglans regia*) [23]. To resolve crystal structure of human tyrosinase, Lai *et al.* [24] have developed expression and purification of human tyrosinase and acquired good crystals of tyrosinase.

3. COMPUTER AIDED METHODS FOR THE IDENTIFICATION OF INHIBITORS OF TYROSINASE

Computational tools have been of much interest in the elucidation and development of new and potent compounds [25]. It has made progress parallel with the advances in bio-molecular spectroscopic practices like XRD (X-ray crystallography), NMR (nuclear magnetic resonance), which enabled great development in the field of molecular biology and structural biology [26]. Computer aided methods offer essential information regarding structure of macromolecular drug targets and have validated three dimensional structure of different proteins [27, 28].

SBDD, structure based drug design is the main factor of medicinal chemistry of modern world. Most often, molecular docking technique of SBDD is used due to its wide range of application in the resolution of various molecular events like molecular interactions, binding energetics and induced conformational changes [29]. Keeping in view of this perception, researchers have introduced *in silico* molecular docking technique for the elucidation of tyrosinase inhibitors. *In silico* docking provides current updates to understand the complex strategies of intermolecular interactions between different chemical analogues and tyrosinase [30].

4. INHIBITORS OF TYROSINASE FROM NATURAL ORIGIN AND THEIR MOLECULAR DOCKING STUDIES

4.1. Arabinose

Arabinose is naturally found in hemicelluloses, pectin and gums. It is five carbon chain monosaccharide with an aldehyde functional group. Arabinose was found to have tyrosinase inhibitory activity. Various polysaccharides and arabinose isolated from *Cuscuta chinensis* was observed to inhibit tyrosinase activity in a mixed type manner *via* down-regulation of tyrosinase expression in B16 melanoma cells [31].

Through kinetic analysis, it was revealed that arabinose facilitated tyrosinase inhibition follows first order kinetics. Molecular docking study between arabinose and tyrosinase showed that HIS61, MET280 and ASN260 were the amino acid residues of tyrosinase with which arabinose binds [32]. Another molecular docking study suggested that D-(-)-arabinose mostly interacts with three histidine residues found in the active site of tyrsoinase (HIS85, HIS259 and HIS263) [33]. These approaches of investigating tyrosinase inhibition by aldehydes and hydroxyl groups through docking simulation may prove potential for finding quite effective tyrosinase inhibitors.

4.2. Hesperitin

Hesperitin is a naturally occurring flavonoid, mostly found in orange and lemon. It was shown to have various therapeutic properties, including antioxidant, anti-inflammation, insulin sensitization, and lipid lowering. Due to this, hesperitinn is used against several ailments such as cardiovascular diseases, psychiatric disorders, neurological disorders and others [34 - 36]. Along with all these properties, hesperitin was also found to have antimelanogenic activity. Findings of Galgut and Ali [37] have observed that glycoside of hesperitin, a hesperidin isolated from citrus peel can stimulate adrenergic receptors present in tail melanocytes of tadpoles resulting into skin lightening effect.

Si *et al.* [38] have successfully simulated tyrosinase and hesperitin using molecular docking algorithms. Their results suggested that hesperitin interacts with amino acid residues including HIS61, HIS85 and HIS259 present at the active site of tyrosinase. It reversibly inhibits tyrosinase in a competitive manner.

4.3. Isorhamnetin

Isorhamnetin belongs to the flavonol class of organic compounds known for its therapeutic properties, including antioxidation [39], cytoprotection [40], anti-atipogenesis [41], and anti-inflammation [42]. Isorhamnetin was observed as an antimelanogenesis agent by Si *et al.* [43] by performing molecular docking between isorhamnetin and tyrosinase. Results of their study showed that isorhamnetin inhibits tyrosinase in a reversible manner. Isorhamnetin was found to interact with various amino acid residues of tyrosinase but more frequently bind with MET280 and HIS244.

4.4. Rutin

Rutin is naturally found in fruits and vegetables. It is also known as quercetin--rutinoside. Buckwheat seeds (*Fagopyrum esculantum*, well known for its anti-diabetic and thrombolytic activity, are found as a rich source of rutin [44 - 46]. Rutin can also act as a depigmentation agent. An *in vitro* study conducted by deFreitas *et al.* [47] using mouse melanoma, human keratinocytes and fibroblast cells have shown that extract of *Morus nigra* leaves standardized in chlorogenic acid, rutin, and isoquercetrin inhibits tyrosinase. Using AutoDock vina software, Si *et al.* [48] have performed docking algorithms between tyrosinase and rutin. Their results suggested that one of the two copper cations present at the active site of tyrosinase was responsible for binding with rutin. Rutin competitively inhibits tyrosinase. Rutin interacts with a number of amino acid residues such as HIS56, HIS80, HIS89, HIS234, HIS249, HIS253, HIS267, HIS281, TYR73, TYR179, LYS74, ALA75, PHE85, PHE269, ASP238, ASP250, ASP266, ASP307, GLU246, PRO268, PHE269 present in tyrosinase.

4.5. Dieckol

Dieckol is mostly present in *Ecklonia cava*, which is a marine algea. It is a hexameric compound of phlorotannin class. It was found to increase hair growth [49] and when mixed with hydrolysate of human placenta it showed antiageing property [50]. Dieckol also exhibits various other therapeutic potentials including anti-proliferative, angio-genic [51], anti-cancer [52] and anti-inflammatory activity [53]. Heo *et al.* [54] have studied the melanogenesis inhibitory effect of dieckol isolated from *Ecklonia cava*. Dieckol was also shown to have protective effect on photooxidative stress induced by UVB radiations. Kang *et al.* [55] have used docking algorithm to found out interaction between dieckol and tyrosinase. Results of their findings suggested that dieckol mostly interacts with HIS208, GLY46 and MET215 amino acid residues of tyrosinase. Dieckol inhibits tyrosinase in a non- competitive way and its property of melanin reduction was found more effective than arbutin, which is a known commercial inhibitor of tyrosinase [55].

4.6. Oxymatrine

Oxymatrine is among the various quinolizidine alkaloid compounds extracted from *Sophora flavescent*, a Chinese herb. It was found to have many therapeutic properties including protection against fibrotic tissue damage, tumor, apoptosis and inflammation [56 - 58]. In addition to these properties, Liu *et al.* [59] have observed its antityrosinase property. They have conducted docking simulation between oxymatrine and tyrosinase using AutoDock 4.2 and Dock 6.3. Their results implied that oxymatrine usually binds with CYS83 and HIS263 amino acod residues present within the active site of tyrosinase. Oxymatrine inhibited tyrosinase in a mixed type manner.

4.7. Morin

3,5,7,2',4'-penta hydroxyl flavone, commonly called morin is a yellow compound of flavonol family. It is naturally found in leaves of guava, onion and seaweeds. It was observed that morin exhibited various therapeutic properties including antibacterial, antioxidant, anti-inflammatory [60] and neuroprotective [61]. Along with other properties, morin was also found to inhibit an enzyme tyrosinase in a competitive manner and hence possess antimelanogenic property [62]. In order to identify the mechanism of tyrosinase inhibition, Wang *et al.* [63] have conducted docking simulation between morin and tyrosinase. They have found that morin bound with HIS85, HIS94, HIS259, HIS263, HIS296, ASN260, PHE264, MET280, GLY281, VAL283 amino acid residues of tyrosinase. Wang *et al.* [63]

further concluded that if foods like leaves of guava and onion, rich in morin are consumed preventing the skin from hyperpigmentation.

4.8. Ascorbic Acid

Ascorbic acid commonly known as vitamin C is found in citrus fruits and tropical fruits. It plays an essential function in human body to keep the teeth, bones, cartilages, skin and blood vessels of the body healthy. Vitamin C prevents our body cells from damage by removing free radicals and acts as an antioxidant [64]. There are various studies which have supported the inhibitory effect of ascorbic acid on the activity of tyrosinase. One such study was conducted by Ros *et al.* [65] in which they have observed the monophenolase activity of tyrosinase using tyrosine as a substrate. No direct effect on tyrosinase with different concentration of ascorbic acid was observed. But, reduction in induction period of hydroxylation of tyrosine was observed.

Senol *et al.* [66] have demonstrated that ascorbic acid inhibits tyrosinase in a remarkable way. They have conducted *in vitro* and *in silico* studies and observed that ascorbic acid is a strong inhibitor of tyrosinase. Molecular docking algorithms and calculations showed that ascorbic acid mostly bind with HIS263, PHE264, SER282 and VAL283 amino acid residue of tyrosinase. Two hydrogen bonds were formed between tyrosinase and ascorbic acids *via* two copper cations of tyrosinase [66].

4.9. Salidroside

Salidroside is a type of flavonoids having phenol glycosides structure. It is an active biocompound of root extracts of *Rhodiola rosea* [67]. Various healing properties like antioxidation [68], anti-inflammation [69], scavenging free radical [70] are found in salidroside. Besides this, it also inhibits enzyme tyrrosinase. Salidroside extracted from the alcoholic extract of *Rhodiola rosea* was found to inhibit melanin synthesis by regulating MITF/CREB/tyrosinase pathway [71]. Zhu *et al.* [72] have conducted docking simulation between tyrosinase and salidroside and showed that salidroside interacts with HIS97, ASN191, ALA202 and THR203 amino acid residues of tyrosinase. Their results suggested that salidroside binds with tyrosinase through bonds which are mostly weak bonds like Vander waal bonds and hydrogen bonds.

4.10. Apigenin

Apigenin (4', 5, 7-trihydroxy flavone) is a flavone naturally found in many plants including parsley, onions, tea, oranges, grapefruit, wheat sprouts, chamomile, *etc.* But, the main source of apigenin is chamomile tea made from the *Matricaria chamomilla*. Apigenin is considered as valuable and health promoting agent as it exhibits various therapeutic properties, including anti-inflammatory, antioxidant, antitumour, anti-depressant, *etc* [73 - 75].

Additionally, it has been found that apigenin inhibits the activity of tyrosinase or polyphenoloxidase. Significant inhibition against mushroom tyrosinase was shown by the apigenin extracted from *Hemisteptia lyrata* [76]. It inhibits tyrosinase reversibly in a mixed type manner. Xiong *et al.* [77] have performed molecular docking between tyrosinase and apigenin using AutoDock Vina and CDocker software to study the mechanism of inhibition. It was found that apigenin is commonly bound with PHE90, VAL248, GLU256 and HIS296 residues of tyrosinase.

4.11. Phloretin

Phloretin, a dihydrochalcone is a type of natural phenol. It is abundantly found in apple, pear, tomato and apricot. It has been found to inhibit the growth of several cancer cells. It is a well known inhibitor of eukaryotic urea transporter, blocks VacA-mediated urea and ion transport [78, 79]. Phloretin is found to inhibit the enzyme tyrosinase, hence it might control the overproduction of melanin. Chen *et al.* [80] have reported that it inhibits tyrosinase in a mixed type manner. They have used AutoDock 4.2.6 to explore the possible interactions between tyrosinase and phloretin. The results showed that phloretin binds to the gate of active site of tyrosinase consist of the two copper cations and His-61, His-85, His-94, His-263 and His-296 amino acid residues. More precisely, phloretin interacts with tyrosinase by three hydrogen bonds with residues Met-280, His-244 and Asn-260 as well as hydrophobic interaction between phloretin and 12 amino acid residues of tyrosinase. Structures of all the compounds discussed above are shown in Fig. (1) and the details of their docking simulation with tyrosinase is presented in Table **1**.

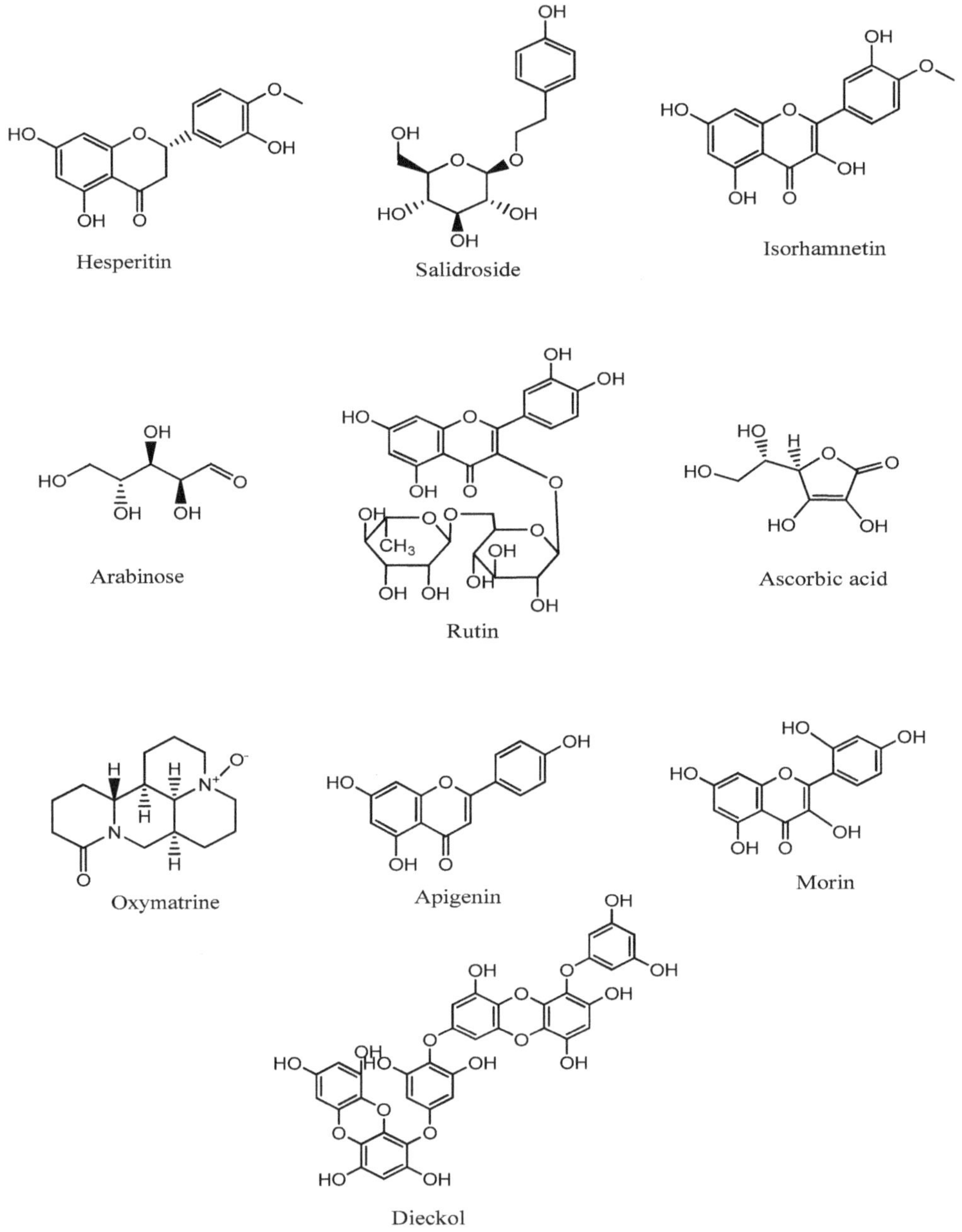

Fig. (1). Chemical structures of the natural compounds having tyrosinase inhibitory activity.

Table 1. Details of the docking simulation between tyrosinase and some natural compounds.

Inhibitors	Tyrosinase (Source organism)	Docking Software Used	Binding Energy/ MolDock Score (Kcal/mol)	Type of Inhibition	References
Hesperitin	*Agaricus bisporus*	Dock 6.3	-34.41	Competitive	[38]
		AutoDock 4.2	-5.61		
Salidroside	*Streptomyces castaneoglobisporus*	AutoDock Vina 1.1.2	NA	Competitive	[72]
Isorhamnetin	*Agaricus bisporus*	Dock 6.3	-32.58	Mixed type	[43]
		AutoDock 4.2	-5.66		
		Fred 2.2	-48.86		
Arabinose	*Agaricus bisporus*	Dock 6.3	-26.28	Mixed type	[32]
		AutoDock 4.2	-2.02		
Rutin	*Agaricus bisporus*	AutoDock Vina	-9.1	Competitive	[48]
Ascorbic acid	*Agaricus bisporus*	Molegro Virtual Docker	-72.63	Mixed type	[66]
Oxymatrine	*Agaricus bisporus*	Dock 6	-118.81	Mixed type	[59]
		AutoDock 4	-8.04		
Apigenin	*Agaricus bisporus*	AutoDock Vina	-8.8	Mixed type	[77]
		CDocker	-38.1		
Morin	*Agaricus bisporus*	AutoDock 4.2	-4.22	Competitive	[63]
Dieckol	*Bacillus megaterium*	CDocker	-126.12	Non-competitive	[55]
Phloretin	*Agaricus bisporus*	AutoDock 4.2.6	-5.32	Mixed type	[80]

5. DESIGN, SYNTHESIS AND ANTITYROSINASE MECHANISM OF DIFFERENT ANALOGUES USING COMPUTATIONAL TOOLS

Development of potent tyrosinase inhibitors is a promising approach to combat skin hyperpigmentation. Hydroxy substituted naphthyl chalcone oxime compounds were synthesized and validated for their antityrosinase activity by using docking algorithm. Two of the synthesized oxime compounds were identified as competitive inhibitors of tyrosinase and found to be twice active than control kojic acid [81]. A series of biphenyl compounds including 2-([1,1--biphenyl]-4-yl)-2-oxoethyl benzoates, 2(a-q), and 2-([1,1'-biphenyl]4yl)-2 oxoethyl pyridinecarboxylate, 2(r-s) were synthesized by reacting various carboxylic acid with 1-([1,1'-biphenyl]-4-yl)-2-bromoethan-1-one using potassium carbonate in dimethylformamide. Among them, five of the compounds were reported to have tyrosinase inhibitory activity, in which 2p, 2r, 2s exhibited more inhibition as compared to the control kojic acid. Computational molecular docking studies further confirmed the results [82]. Similarly a series of 1-pentanoyl-3-arylthioureas were designed and synthesized for their antityrosinase activity. Structure of them was identified and confirmed by the state of the art techniques of NMR, FTIR, XRD. Results of docking studies of all compounds showed that compound 4(f) exhibited more inhibitory activity as it showed highest affinity with tyrosinase [83].

Recently, Butt *et al.* [84] have synthesized novel bi-heterocyclic acetamides 9a-n. All these compounds were detected as potent tyrosinase inhibitors by using enzyme kinetics and computational studies. Similarly, Karakaya *et al.* [85] have synthesized kojic acid derivatives and their efficacy for tyrosinase inhibition was confirmed by molecular docking analysis. In a recent study by Iraji *et al.* [86] synthesized 4 hydroxy-N'-methylenebenzohydrazide derivatives and evaluated their tyrosinase inhibitory activity by using molecular docking algorithms. So, they concluded that these derivatives can be used as potent antimelanogenic agents for the treatment of hyperpgmentation [86]. Very recently, Nazir *et al.* [87] have synthesized (2-(3-methoxyphenoxy)-2-oxoethyl (E)-3-(4-hydroxyphenyl) acrylate) and (2-(3-methoxyphenoxy)-2-oxoethyl 2, 4-dihydroxybenzoate). Both the compounds showed tyrosinase inhibitory activity as revealed by docking of these compounds with tyrosinase.

CONCLUSION

Melasma, ephelides, solar lentigines, *etc.* are the various forms of skin hyperpig-mentation caused by the excess production of melanin. Tyrosinase is the key enzyme of melanin synthesis. Hence the search for the inhibitors of tyrosinase is an important target to facilitate the development of therapies for skin hyperpig-mentation. Besides *in vitro* and *in vivo* methods, *in silico* methods have proven very useful to evaluate tyrosinase inhibitors. Through molecular docking approach, intermolecular interaction of tyrosinase with the inhibitors has been predicted. Thus, further research breakthrough with the aid of computational biology and chemistry, more precisely bioinformatics, will bring new hope in the development of potent inhibitors of tyrsoinase that will eventually benefit people to get relief from the hyper pigmentary disorders.

REFERENCES

[1]　Chang, T.S. An updated review of tyrosinase inhibitors. *Int. J. Mol. Sci.,* **2009**, *10*(6), 2440-2475.
[http://dx.doi.org/10.3390/ijms10062440] [PMID: 19582213]

[2]　Mapunya, M.B.; Nikolova, R.V.; Lall, N. Melanogenesis and antityrosinase activity of selected South african plants. *Evid. Based Complement. Alternat. Med.,* **2012**, *2012*, 374017.
[http://dx.doi.org/10.1155/2012/374017] [PMID: 22611429]

[3]　Visscher, M.O. Skin color and pigmentation in ethnic skin. *Facial Plast. Surg. Clin. North Am.,* **2017**, *25*(1), 119-125.
[http://dx.doi.org/10.1016/j.fsc.2016.08.011] [PMID: 27888889]

[4]　Kim, Y.J.; Uyama, H. Tyrosinase inhibitors from natural and synthetic sources: structure, inhibition mechanism and perspective for the future. *Cell. Mol. Life Sci.,* **2005**, *62*(15), 1707-1723.
[http://dx.doi.org/10.1007/s00018-005-5054-y] [PMID: 15968468]

[5]　Khan, M.T. Novel tyrosinase inhibitors from natural resources - their computational studies. *Curr. Med. Chem.,* **2012**, *19*(14), 2262-2272.
[http://dx.doi.org/10.2174/092986712800229041] [PMID: 22414108]

[6]　Jia, Y.L.; Zheng, J.; Yu, F.; Cai, Y.X.; Zhan, X.L.; Wang, H.F.; Chen, Q.X. Anti-tyrosinase kinetics and antibacterial process of caffeic acid N-nonyl ester in Chinese Olive (*Canarium album*) postharvest. *Int. J. Biol. Macromol.,* **2016**, *91*, 486-495.
[http://dx.doi.org/10.1016/j.ijbiomac.2016.05.098] [PMID: 27246378]

[7]　Parvez, S.; Kang, M.; Chung, H.S.; Bae, H. Naturally occurring tyrosinase inhibitors: mechanism and applications in skin health, cosmetics and agriculture industries. *Phytother. Res.,* **2007**, *21*(9), 805-816.
[http://dx.doi.org/10.1002/ptr.2184] [PMID: 17605157]

[8]　Asadzadeh, A.; Sirous, H.; Pourfarzam, M.; Yaghmaei, P.; Afshin, F. *In vitro* and *in silico* studies of the inhibitory effects of some novel kojic acid derivatives on tyrosinase enzyme. *Iran. J. Basic Med. Sci.,* **2016**, *19*(2), 132-144.
[PMID: 27081457]

[9]　Jorgensen, W.L. Efficient drug lead discovery and optimization. *Acc. Chem. Res.,* **2009**, *42*(6), 724-733.
[http://dx.doi.org/10.1021/ar800236t] [PMID: 19317443]

[10]　Clark, D.E. What has virtual screening ever done for drug discovery? *Expert Opin. Drug Discov.,* **2008**, *3*(8), 841-851.
[http://dx.doi.org/10.1517/17460441.3.8.841] [PMID: 23484962]

[11]　Issa, N.T.; Wathieu, H.; Ojo, A.; Byers, S.W.; Dakshanamurthy, S. Drug metabolism in preclinical drug development: A survey of the discovery process, toxicology, and computational tools. *Curr. Drug Metab.,* **2017**, *18*(6), 556-565.
[http://dx.doi.org/10.2174/1389200218666170316093301] [PMID: 28302026]

[12]　Chase, M.R.; Raina, K.; Bruno, J.; Sugumaran, M. Purification, characterization and molecular cloning of prophenoloxidases from *Sarcophaga bullata*. *Insect Biochem. Mol. Biol.,* **2000**, *30*(10), 953-967.
[http://dx.doi.org/10.1016/S0965-1748(00)00068-0] [PMID: 10899462]

[13]　Oetting, W.S. The tyrosinase gene and oculocutaneous albinism type 1 (OCA1): A model for understanding the molecular biology of melanin formation. *Pigment Cell Res.,* **2000**, *13*(5), 320-325.
[http://dx.doi.org/10.1034/j.1600-0749.2000.130503.x] [PMID: 11041207]

[14]　Zaidi, K.U.; Ali, S.A.; Ali, A.S. Melanogenic effect of purified mushroom tyrosinase on B16F10 Melanocytes: A Phase Contrast and Immunofluorescence Microscopic Study. *J Microsc Ultrastruct,* **2017**, *5*(2), 82-89.
[http://dx.doi.org/10.1016/j.jmau.2016.07.002] [PMID: 30023240]

[15]　Cooksey, C.J.; Garratt, P.J.; Land, E.J.; Pavel, S.; Ramsden, C.A.; Riley, P.A.; Smit, N.P.M. Evidence of the indirect formation of the catecholic intermediate substrate responsible for the autoactivation

kinetics of tyrosinase. *J. Biol. Chem.*, **1997**, *272*(42), 26226-26235.
[http://dx.doi.org/10.1074/jbc.272.42.26226] [PMID: 9334191]

[16]   Kumar, C.M.; Sathisha, U.V.; Dharmesh, S.; Rao, A.G.; Singh, S.A. Interaction of sesamol (3,4-methylenedioxyphenol) with tyrosinase and its effect on melanin synthesis. *Biochimie*, **2011**, *93*(3), 562-569.
[http://dx.doi.org/10.1016/j.biochi.2010.11.014] [PMID: 21144881]

[17]   Solomon, E.I.; Sundaram, U.M.; Machonkin, T.E. Multicopper oxidases and oxygenases. *Chem. Rev.*, **1996**, *96*(7), 2563-2606.
[http://dx.doi.org/10.1021/cr950046o] [PMID: 11848837]

[18]   Lind, T.; Siegbahn, P.E.M.; Crabtree, R.H. A quantum chemical study of the mechanism of tyrosinase. *J. Phys. Chem.*, **1999**, *103*(7), 1193-1202.
[http://dx.doi.org/10.1021/jp982321r]

[19]   Decker, H.; Tuczek, F. Tyrosinase/catecholoxidase activity of hemocyanins: structural basis and molecular mechanism. *Trends Biochem. Sci.*, **2000**, *25*(8), 392-397.
[http://dx.doi.org/10.1016/S0968-0004(00)01602-9] [PMID: 10916160]

[20]   Matoba, Y.; Kumagai, T.; Yamamoto, A.; Yoshitsu, H.; Sugiyama, M. Crystallographic evidence that the dinuclear copper center of tyrosinase is flexible during catalysis. *J. Biol. Chem.*, **2006**, *281*(13), 8981-8990.
[http://dx.doi.org/10.1074/jbc.M509785200] [PMID: 16436386]

[21]   Sendovski, M.; Kanteev, M.; Ben-Yosef, V.S.; Adir, N.; Fishman, A. First structures of an active bacterial tyrosinase reveal copper plasticity. *J. Mol. Biol.*, **2011**, *405*(1), 227-237.
[http://dx.doi.org/10.1016/j.jmb.2010.10.048] [PMID: 21040728]

[22]   Ismaya, W.T.; Rozeboom, H.J.; Weijn, A.; Mes, J.J.; Fusetti, F.; Wichers, H.J.; Dijkstra, B.W. Crystal structure of *Agaricus bisporus* mushroom tyrosinase: identity of the tetramer subunits and interaction with tropolone. *Biochemistry*, **2011**, *50*(24), 5477-5486.
[http://dx.doi.org/10.1021/bi200395t] [PMID: 21598903]

[23]   Bijelic, A.; Pretzler, M.; Molitor, C.; Zekiri, F.; Rompel, A. The Structure of a plant tyrosinase from walnut leaves reveals the importance of "Substrate-guiding residues" for enzymatic specificity. *Angew. Chem. Int. Ed. Engl.*, **2015**, *54*(49), 14677-14680.
[http://dx.doi.org/10.1002/anie.201506994] [PMID: 26473311]

[24]   Lai, X.; Soler-Lopez, M.; Wichers, H.J.; Dijkstra, B.W. Large-scale recombinant expression and purification of human tyrosinase suitable for structural studies. *PLoS One*, **2016**, *11*(8), e0161697.
[http://dx.doi.org/10.1371/journal.pone.0161697] [PMID: 27551823]

[25]   Greer, J.; Erickson, J.W.; Baldwin, J.J.; Varney, M.D. Application of the three-dimensional structures of protein target molecules in structure-based drug design. *J. Med. Chem.*, **1994**, *37*(8), 1035-1054.
[http://dx.doi.org/10.1021/jm00034a001] [PMID: 8164249]

[26]   Müller, B.A. Imatinib and its successors--how modern chemistry has changed drug development. *Curr. Pharm. Des.*, **2009**, *15*(2), 120-133.
[http://dx.doi.org/10.2174/138161209787002933] [PMID: 19149608]

[27]   Salum, L.B.; Polikarpov, I.; Andricopulo, A.D. Structure-based approach for the study of estrogen receptor binding affinity and subtype selectivity. *J. Chem. Inf. Model.*, **2008**, *48*(11), 2243-2253.
[http://dx.doi.org/10.1021/ci8002182] [PMID: 18937440]

[28]   McRobb, F.M.; Negri, A.; Beuming, T.; Sherman, W. Molecular dynamics techniques for modeling G protein-coupled receptors. *Curr. Opin. Pharmacol.*, **2016**, *30*, 69-75.
[http://dx.doi.org/10.1016/j.coph.2016.07.001] [PMID: 27490828]

[29]   Weigelt, J. Structural genomics-impact on biomedicine and drug discovery. *Exp. Cell Res.*, **2010**, *316*(8), 1332-1338.
[http://dx.doi.org/10.1016/j.yexcr.2010.02.041] [PMID: 20211166]

[30]   Cheng, M.; Chen, Z. Screening of tyrosinase inhibitors by capillary electrophoresis with immobilized enzyme microreactor and molecular docking. *Electrophoresis,* **2017**, *38*(3-4), 486-493.
[http://dx.doi.org/10.1002/elps.201600367] [PMID: 27862041]

[31]   Liu, Z.J.; Wang, Y.L.; Li, Q.L.; Yang, L. Improved antimelanogenesis and antioxidant effects of polysaccharide from *Cuscuta chinensis* Lam seeds after enzymatic hydrolysis. *Braz. J. Med. Biol. Res.,* **2018**, *51*(7), e7256.
[http://dx.doi.org/10.1590/1414-431x20187256] [PMID: 29846408]

[32]   Hu, W.J.; Yan, L.; Park, D.; Jeong, H.O.; Chung, H.Y.; Yang, J.M.; Ye, Z.M.; Qian, G.Y. Kinetic, structural and molecular docking studies on the inhibition of tyrosinase induced by arabinose. *Int. J. Biol. Macromol.,* **2012**, *50*(3), 694-700.
[http://dx.doi.org/10.1016/j.ijbiomac.2011.12.035] [PMID: 22245359]

[33]   Liu, H.J.; Ji, S.; Fan, Y.Q.; Yan, L.; Yang, J.M.; Zhou, H.M.; Lee, J.; Wang, Y.L. The effect of D-(−-arabinose on tyrosinase: an integrated study using computational simulation and inhibition kinetics. *Enzyme Res,* **2012**, *2012*(2012), 1-10.

[34]   Akiyama, S.; Katsumata, S.; Suzuki, K.; Nakaya, Y.; Ishimi, Y.; Uehara, M. Hypoglycemic and hypolipidemic effects of hesperidin and cyclodextrin-clathrated hesperetin in Goto-Kakizaki rats with type 2 diabetes. *Biosci. Biotechnol. Biochem.,* **2009**, *73*(12), 2779-2782.
[http://dx.doi.org/10.1271/bbb.90576] [PMID: 19966469]

[35]   Ahmed, O.M.; Mahmoud, A.M.; Abdel-Moneim, A.; Ashour, M.B. Antidiabetic effects of hesperidin and naringin in type 2 diabetic rats. *Diabetol. Croat.,* **2012**, *41*(2), 53-67.

[36]   Li, C.; Schluesener, H. Health-promoting effects of the citrus flavanone hesperidin. *Crit. Rev. Food Sci. Nutr.,* **2017**, *57*(3), 613-631.
[http://dx.doi.org/10.1080/10408398.2014.906382] [PMID: 25675136]

[37]   Galgut, J.M.; Ali, S.A. Hesperidin induced melanophore aggregatory responses in tadpole of Bufo melanostictus *via* α- Adrenoceptors. *Pharmacologia,* **2012**, *3*(10), 519-524.
[http://dx.doi.org/10.5567/pharmacologia.2012.519.524]

[38]   Si, Y.X.; Wang, Z.J.; Park, D.; Chung, H.Y.; Wang, S.F.; Yan, L.; Yang, J.M.; Qian, G.Y.; Yin, S.J.; Park, Y.D. Effect of hesperetin on tyrosinase: inhibition kinetics integrated computational simulation study. *Int. J. Biol. Macromol.,* **2012**, *50*(1), 257-262.
[http://dx.doi.org/10.1016/j.ijbiomac.2011.11.001] [PMID: 22093614]

[39]   Pengfei, L.; Tiansheng, D.; Xianglin, H.; Jianguo, W. Antioxidant properties of isolated isorhamnetin from the sea buckthorn marc. *Plant Foods Hum. Nutr.,* **2009**, *64*(2), 141-145.
[http://dx.doi.org/10.1007/s11130-009-0116-1] [PMID: 19444611]

[40]   Upadhyay, N.K.; Kumar, M.S.; Gupta, A. Antioxidant, cytoprotective and antibacterial effects of Sea buckthorn (*Hippophae rhamnoides* L.) leaves. *Food Chem. Toxicol.,* **2010**, *48*(12), 3443-3448.
[http://dx.doi.org/10.1016/j.fct.2010.09.019] [PMID: 20854873]

[41]   Lee, J.; Lee, J.; Jung, E.; Hwang, W.; Kim, Y.S.; Park, D. Isorhamnetin-induced anti-adipogenesis is mediated by stabilization of beta-catenin protein. *Life Sci.,* **2010**, *86*(11-12), 416-423.
[http://dx.doi.org/10.1016/j.lfs.2010.01.012] [PMID: 20097210]

[42]   Hämäläinen, M.; Nieminen, R.; Asmawi, M.Z.; Vuorela, P.; Vapaatalo, H.; Moilanen, E. Effects of flavonoids on prostaglandin E2 production and on COX-2 and mPGES-1 expressions in activated macrophages. *Planta Med.,* **2011**, *77*(13), 1504-1511.
[http://dx.doi.org/10.1055/s-0030-1270762] [PMID: 21341175]

[43]   Si, Y.X.; Wang, Z.J.; Park, D.; Jeong, H.O.; Ye, S.; Chung, H.Y.; Yang, J.M.; Yin, S.J.; Qian, G.Y. Effects of isorhamnetin on tyrosinase: inhibition kinetics and computational simulation. *Biosci. Biotechnol. Biochem.,* **2012**, *76*(6), 1091-1097.
[http://dx.doi.org/10.1271/bbb.110910] [PMID: 22790928]

[44]   Bai, C.Z.; Feng, M.L.; Hao, X.L.; Zhong, Q.M.; Tong, L.G.; Wang, Z.H. Rutin, quercetin, and free

amino acid analysis in buckwheat (*Fagopyrum*) seeds from different locations. *Genet. Mol. Res.,* **2015**, *14*(4), 19040-19048.
[http://dx.doi.org/10.4238/2015.December.29.11] [PMID: 26782554]

[45]   Sattanathan, K.; Dhanapal, C.K.; Umarani, R.; Manavalan, R. Beneficial health effects of rutin supplementation in patients with diabetes mellitus. *J. Appl. Pharm. Sci.,* **2011**, *1*(8), 227-231.

[46]   Dar, M. A and Tabassum, N. Rutin-potent thrombolytic agent. *Int. Curr. Pharm. J.,* **2012**, *1*(12), 431-435.
[http://dx.doi.org/10.3329/icpj.v1i12.12454]

[47]   de Freitas, M.M.; Fontes, P.R.; Souza, P.M.; William Fagg, C.; Neves Silva Guerra, E.; de Medeiros Nóbrega, Y.K.; Silveira, D.; Fonseca-Bazzo, Y.; Simeoni, L.A.; Homem-de-Mello, M.; Oliveira Magalhães, P. Extracts of Morus nigra L. Leaves Standardized in Chlorogenic Acid, Rutin and Isoquercitrin: Tyrosinase Inhibition and Cytotoxicity. *PLoS One,* **2016**, *11*(9), e0163130.
[http://dx.doi.org/10.1371/journal.pone.0163130] [PMID: 27655047]

[48]   Si, Y.X.; Yin, S.J.; Oh, S.; Wang, Z.J.; Ye, S.; Yan, L.; Yang, J.M.; Park, Y.D.; Lee, J.; Qian, G.Y. An integrated study of tyrosinase inhibition by rutin: progress using a computational simulation. *J. Biomol. Struct. Dyn.,* **2012**, *29*(5), 999-1012.
[http://dx.doi.org/10.1080/073911012010525028] [PMID: 22292957]

[49]   Kang, J.I.; Kim, S.C.; Kim, M.K.; Boo, H.J.; Jeon, Y.J.; Koh, Y.S.; Yoo, E.S.; Kang, S.M.; Kang, H.K. Effect of Dieckol, a component of Ecklonia cava, on the promotion of hair growth. *Int. J. Mol. Sci.,* **2012**, *13*(5), 6407-6423.
[http://dx.doi.org/10.3390/ijms13056407] [PMID: 22754373]

[50]   Jang, S.K.; Lee, D.I.; Kim, S.T.; Kim, G.H.; Park, W.; Park, J.Y.; Han, D.; Choi, J.K.; Lee, Y.B.; Han, N.S.; Kim, Y.B.; Han, J.; Joo, S.S. The anti-aging properties of a human placental hydrolysate combined with dieckol isolated from Ecklonia cava. *BMC Complement. Altern. Med.,* **2015**, *15*, 345.
[http://dx.doi.org/10.1186/s12906-015-0876-0] [PMID: 26438076]

[51]   Li, Y.X.; Li, Y.; Je, J.Y.; Kim, S.K. Dieckol as a novel anti-proliferative and anti-angiogenic agent and computational anti-angiogenic activity evaluation. *Environ. Toxicol. Pharmacol.,* **2015**, *39*(1), 259-270.
[http://dx.doi.org/10.1016/j.etap.2014.11.027] [PMID: 25531264]

[52]   Jeong, S.H.; Jeon, Y.J.; Park, S.J. Inhibitory effects of dieckol on hypoxia-induced epithelial-mesenchymal transition of HT29 human colorectal cancer cells. *Mol. Med. Rep.,* **2016**, *14*(6), 5148-5154.
[http://dx.doi.org/10.3892/mmr.2016.5872] [PMID: 27779676]

[53]   Yang, Y.I.; Woo, J.H.; Seo, Y.J.; Lee, K.T.; Lim, Y.; Choi, J.H. Protective effect of brown alga phlorotannins against hyper-inflammatory responses in lipopolysaccharide-induced sepsis models. *J. Agric. Food Chem.,* **2016**, *64*(3), 570-578.
[http://dx.doi.org/10.1021/acs.jafc.5b04482] [PMID: 26730445]

[54]   Heo, S.J.; Ko, S.C.; Cha, S.H.; Kang, D.H.; Park, H.S.; Choi, Y.U.; Kim, D.; Jung, W.K.; Jeon, Y.J. Effect of phlorotannins isolated from Ecklonia cava on melanogenesis and their protective effect against photo-oxidative stress induced by UV-B radiation. *Toxicol. In Vitro,* **2009**, *23*(6), 1123-1130.
[http://dx.doi.org/10.1016/j.tiv.2009.05.013] [PMID: 19490939]

[55]   Kang, S.M.; Heo, S.J.; Kim, K.N.; Lee, S.H.; Yang, H.M.; Kim, A.D.; Jeon, Y.J. Molecular docking studies of a phlorotannin, dieckol isolated from *Ecklonia cava* with tyrosinase inhibitory activity. *Bioorg. Med. Chem.,* **2012**, *20*(1), 311-316.
[http://dx.doi.org/10.1016/j.bmc.2011.10.078] [PMID: 22112542]

[56]   Yamazaki, M. The pharmacological studies on matrine and oxymatrine. *Yakugaku Zasshi,* **2000**, *120*(10), 1025-1033.
[http://dx.doi.org/10.1248/yakushi1947.120.10_1025] [PMID: 11082713]

[57]   Ma, L.; Wen, S.; Zhan, Y.; He, Y.; Liu, X.; Jiang, J. Anticancer effects of the Chinese medicine

matrine on murine hepatocellular carcinoma cells. *Planta Med.,* **2008**, *74*(3), 245-251.
[http://dx.doi.org/10.1055/s-2008-1034304] [PMID: 18283616]

[58]   Zhang, X.; Jiang, W.; Zhou, A.L.; Zhao, M.; Jiang, D.R. Inhibitory effect of oxymatrine on hepatocyte apoptosis *via* TLR4/PI3K/Akt/GSK-3β signaling pathway. *World J. Gastroenterol.,* **2017**, *23*(21), 3839-3849.
[http://dx.doi.org/10.3748/wjg.v23.i21.3839] [PMID: 28638224]

[59]   Liu, X.X.; Sun, S.Q.; Wang, Y.J.; Xu, W.; Wang, Y.F.; Park, D.; Zhou, H.M.; Han, H.Y. Kinetics and computational docking studies on the inhibition of tyrosinase induced by oxymatrine. *Appl. Biochem. Biotechnol.,* **2013**, *169*(1), 145-158.
[http://dx.doi.org/10.1007/s12010-012-9960-9] [PMID: 23160948]

[60]   Fang, S.H.; Hou, Y.C.; Chang, W.C.; Hsiu, S.L.; Chao, P.D.; Chiang, B.L. Morin sulfates/glucuronides exert anti-inflammatory activity on activated macrophages and decreased the incidence of septic shock. *Life Sci.,* **2003**, *74*(6), 743-756.
[http://dx.doi.org/10.1016/j.lfs.2003.07.017] [PMID: 14654167]

[61]   Lee, K.M.; Lee, Y.; Chun, H.J.; Kim, A.H.; Kim, J.Y.; Lee, J.Y.; Ishigami, A.; Lee, J. Neuroprotective and anti-inflammatory effects of morin in a murine model of Parkinson's disease. *J. Neurosci. Res.,* **2016**, *94*(10), 865-878.
[http://dx.doi.org/10.1002/jnr.23764] [PMID: 27265894]

[62]   Xie, L.P.; Chen, Q.X.; Huang, H.; Wang, H.Z.; Zhang, R.Q. Inhibitory effects of some flavonoids on the activity of mushroom tyrosinase. *Biochemistry (Mosc.),* **2003**, *68*(4), 487-491.
[http://dx.doi.org/10.1023/A:1023620501702] [PMID: 12765534]

[63]   Wang, Y.; Zhang, G.; Yan, J.; Gong, D. Inhibitory effect of morin on tyrosinase: insights from spectroscopic and molecular docking studies. *Food Chem.,* **2014**, *163*, 226-233.
[http://dx.doi.org/10.1016/j.foodchem.2014.04.106] [PMID: 24912720]

[64]   Arrigoni, O.; De Tullio, M.C. Ascorbic acid: much more than just an antioxidant. *Biochim. Biophys. Acta,* **2002**, *1569*(1-3), 1-9.
[http://dx.doi.org/10.1016/S0304-4165(01)00235-5] [PMID: 11853951]

[65]   Ros, J.R.; Rodríguez-López, J.N.; García-Cánovas, F. Effect of L-ascorbic acid on the monophenolase activity of tyrosinase. *Biochem. J.,* **1993**, *295*(Pt 1), 309-312.
[http://dx.doi.org/10.1042/bj2950309] [PMID: 8216233]

[66]   Senol, F.S.; Khan, M.T.; Orhan, G.; Gurkas, E.; Orhan, I.E.; Oztekin, N.S.; Ak, F. In silico approach to inhibition of tyrosinase by ascorbic acid using molecular docking simulations. *Curr. Top. Med. Chem.,* **2014**, *14*(12), 1469-1472.
[http://dx.doi.org/10.2174/1568026614666140610121253] [PMID: 24917394]

[67]   Chen, S.F.; Tsai, H.J.; Hung, T.H.; Chen, C.C.; Lee, C.Y.; Wu, C.H.; Wang, P.Y.; Liao, N.C. Salidroside improves behavioral and histological outcomes and reduces apoptosis *via* PI3K/Akt signaling after experimental traumatic brain injury. *PLoS One,* **2012**, *7*(9), e45763.
[http://dx.doi.org/10.1371/journal.pone.0045763] [PMID: 23029230]

[68]   Kucinskaite, A.; Briedis, V.; Savickas, A. [Experimental analysis of therapeutic properties of *Rhodiola rosea* L. and its possible application in medicine]. *Medicina (Kaunas),* **2004**, *40*(7), 614-619.
[PMID: 15252224]

[69]   Kang, H.S.; Kim, H.R.; Byun, D.S.; Son, B.W.; Nam, T.J.; Choi, J.S. Tyrosinase inhibitors isolated from the edible brown alga *Ecklonia stolonifera*. *Arch. Pharm. Res.,* **2004**, *27*(12), 1226-1232.
[http://dx.doi.org/10.1007/BF02975886] [PMID: 15646796]

[70]   Zhong, H.; Xin, H.; Wu, L.X.; Zhu, Y.Z. Salidroside attenuates apoptosis in ischemic cardiomyocytes: a mechanism through a mitochondria-dependent pathway. *J. Pharmacol. Sci.,* **2010**, *114*(4), 399-408.
[http://dx.doi.org/10.1254/jphs.10078FP] [PMID: 21160132]

[71]   Chiang, H.M.; Chien, Y.C.; Wu, C.H.; Kuo, Y.H.; Wu, W.C.; Pan, Y.Y.; Su, Y.H.; Wen, K.C.

Hydroalcoholic extract of *Rhodiola rosea* L. (Crassulaceae) and its hydrolysate inhibit melanogenesis in B16F0 cells by regulating the CREB/MITF/tyrosinase pathway. *Food Chem. Toxicol.,* **2014**, *65*, 129-139.
[http://dx.doi.org/10.1016/j.fct.2013.12.032] [PMID: 24380755]

[72] Zhu, Y.; Chen, C.; Zhao, S.; Yang, J.; Song, H.; Ge, F.; Liu, D. Inhibitory mechanism of salidroside on tyrosinase. *J. Food Nutr. Res.,* **2014**, *2*(10), 698-703.
[http://dx.doi.org/10.12691/jfnr-2-10-8]

[73] McKay, D.L.; Blumberg, J.B. A review of the bioactivity and potential health benefits of chamomile tea (*Matricaria recutita* L.). *Phytother. Res.,* **2006**, *20*(7), 519-530.
[http://dx.doi.org/10.1002/ptr.1900] [PMID: 16628544]

[74] Li, R.; Zhao, D.; Qu, R.; Fu, Q.; Ma, S. The effects of apigenin on lipopolysaccharide-induced depressive-like behavior in mice. *Neurosci. Lett.,* **2015**, *594*, 17-22.
[http://dx.doi.org/10.1016/j.neulet.2015.03.040] [PMID: 25800110]

[75] Park, S.; Lim, W.; Bazer, F.W.; Song, G. Apigenin induces ROS-dependent apoptosis and ER stress in human endometriosis cells. *J. Cell. Physiol.,* **2018**, *233*(4), 3055-3065.
[http://dx.doi.org/10.1002/jcp.26054] [PMID: 28617956]

[76] Ha, T.J.; Hwang, S.W.; Jung, H.J.; Park, K.H.; Yang, M.S. Apigenin, Tyrosinase Inhibitor Isolated from the Flowers of *Hemisteptia lyrata* Bunge. *J. Korean Soc. Appl. Biol. Chem.,* **2002**, *45*(4), 170-172.

[77] Xiong, Z.; Liu, W.; Zhou, L.; Zou, L.; Chen, J. Mushroom (*Agaricus bisporus*) polyphenoloxidase inhibited by apigenin: Multi-spectroscopic analyses and computational docking simulation. *Food Chem.,* **2016**, *203*, 430-439.
[http://dx.doi.org/10.1016/j.foodchem.2016.02.045] [PMID: 26948635]

[78] Chou, C.L.; Knepper, M.A. Inhibition of urea transport in inner medullary collecting duct by phloretin and urea analogues. *Am. J. Physiol.,* **1989**, *257*(3 Pt 2), F359-F365.
[PMID: 2506765]

[79] Verkman, A.S.; Esteva-Font, C.; Cil, O.; Anderson, M.O.; Li, F.; Li, M.; Lei, T.; Ren, H.; Yang, B. Small-molecule inhibitors of urea transporters. *Subcell. Biochem.,* **2014**, *73*, 165-177.
[http://dx.doi.org/10.1007/978-94-017-9343-8_11] [PMID: 25298345]

[80] Chen, J.; Li, Q.; Ye, Y.; Huang, Z.; Ruan, Z.; Jin, N. Phloretin as both a substrate and inhibitor of tyrosinase: Inhibitory activity and mechanism. *Spectrochim. Acta A Mol. Biomol. Spectrosc.,* **2020**, *226*, 117642.
[http://dx.doi.org/10.1016/j.saa.2019.117642] [PMID: 31614273]

[81] Radhakrishnan, S.; Shimmon, R.; Conn, C.; Baker, A. Integrated kinetic studies and computational analysis on naphthyl chalcones as mushroom tyrosinase inhibitors. *Bioorg. Med. Chem. Lett.,* **2015**, *25*(19), 4085-4091.
[http://dx.doi.org/10.1016/j.bmcl.2015.08.033] [PMID: 26318997]

[82] Kwong, H.C.; Chidan Kumar, C.S.; Mah, S.H.; Chia, T.S.; Quah, C.K.; Loh, Z.H.; Chandraju, S.; Lim, G.K. Novel biphenyl ester derivatives as tyrosinase inhibitors: Synthesis, crystallographic, spectral analysis and molecular docking studies. *PLoS One,* **2017**, *12*(2), e0170117.
[http://dx.doi.org/10.1371/journal.pone.0170117] [PMID: 28241010]

[83] Larik, F.A.; Saeed, A.; Channar, P.A.; Muqadar, U.; Abbas, Q.; Hassan, M.; Seo, S.Y.; Bolte, M. Design, synthesis, kinetic mechanism and molecular docking studies of novel 1-pentanoyl-3-arylthioureas as inhibitors of mushroom tyrosinase and free radical scavengers. *Eur. J. Med. Chem.,* **2017**, *141*, 273-281.
[http://dx.doi.org/10.1016/j.ejmech.2017.09.059] [PMID: 29040952]

[84] Butt, A.R.S.; Abbasi, M.A.; Aziz-Ur-Rehman, ; Siddiqui, S.Z.; Raza, H.; Hassan, M.; Shah, S.A.A.; Shahid, M.; Seo, S.Y. Synthesis and structure-activity relationship of tyrosinase inhibiting novel bi-heterocyclic acetamides: Mechanistic insights through enzyme inhibition, kinetics and computational

studies. *Bioorg. Chem.,* **2019**, *86*, 459-472.
[http://dx.doi.org/10.1016/j.bioorg.2019.01.036] [PMID: 30772647]

[85] Karakaya, G.; Türe, A.; Ercan, A.; Öncül, S.; Aytemir, M.D. Synthesis, computational molecular docking analysis and effectiveness on tyrosinase inhibition of kojic acid derivatives. *Bioorg. Chem.,* **2019**, 102950.
[http://dx.doi.org/10.1016/j.bioorg.2019.102950] [PMID: 31075740]

[86] Iraji, A.; Khoshneviszadeh, M.; Bakhshizadeh, P.; Edraki, N.; Khoshneviszadeh, M. Structure-Based Design, Synthesis, Biological Evaluation and Molecular Docking Study of 4-Hydroxy--'-methylenebenzohydrazide Derivatives Acting as Tyrosinase Inhibitors as Potentiate Anti-Melanogenesis Activities. *Med. Chem.,* **2019**.
[http://dx.doi.org/10.2174/1573406415666190724142951] [PMID: 31339074]

[87] Nazir, Y.; Saeed, A.; Rafiq, M.; Afzal, S.; Ali, A.; Latif, M.; Zuegg, J.; Hussein, W.M.; Fercher, C.; Barnard, R.T.; Cooper, M.A.; Blaskovich, M.A.T.; Ashraf, Z.; Ziora, Z.M. Hydroxyl substituted benzoic acid/cinnamic acid derivatives: Tyrosinase inhibitory kinetics, anti-melanogenic activity and molecular docking studies. *Bioorg. Med. Chem. Lett.,* **2020**, *30*(1), 126722.
[http://dx.doi.org/10.1016/j.bmcl.2019.126722] [PMID: 31732410]

CHAPTER 10

A Preventive Approach to Hypopigmentation and Hyperpigmentation

Abstract: A less or excess production and distribution of melanin pigment leads to pigmentary disorders in human beings. Reduced melanin production results in hypopigmentation, whereas its excess production results in hyperpigmentation. There are several intrinsic and extrinsic factors that are responsible for causing these disorders. Many proteins and enzymes are involved in the complex process of pigmentation called melanogenesis. Any defect in the proteins or enzymes and/or any pathway of melanogenesis due to any of the factors may cause pigmentary disorders. There are certain things that have to be taken care of in order to avoid the dysfunctioning of the components of melanogenesis. Such things include some drugs, chemical reagents, hair dyes, food allergens, prolonged use of antibiotics, use of certain natural allergens, excessive sun exposure *etc*. The present chapter is dedicated to the effects of these things on skin pigmentation and the preventive approach to overcome the problems of skin hypopigmentation and hyperpigmentation caused by them.

Keywords : Food allergens, Melanin, Melanogenesis, Pigmentary disorders, Sun exposure.

1. INTRODUCTION

Melanin is the chief determinant of skin, hair and eye color. Besides this, it plays a crucial role in the protection of the skin against photocarcinogenesis caused by UV radiation. Melanin is produced inside the specialized organelles, melanosomes by the melanocytes in a complex process called melanogenesis [1]. When melanogenesis gets disturbed, it determines different types of pigmentation defects. These defects are classified as hypopigmentation and hyperpigmentation which may occur due to less or excessive melanin production and distribution. This improper production of melanin is caused by several intrinsic and extrinsic factors. Vitiligo, melasma, post inflammatory hyperpigmentation, ephelides, solar lentigines, melasma *etc*. are the various forms of pigmentary disorders [2, 3].

Several enzymes, transcription factors, and other proteins are engaged in melanin synthesis during the process of melanogenesis. Certain substances like antibiotics and other drugs, hair dyes, cosmetics, physiotherapy, food allergens *etc*. can also

Sharique A. Ali & Naima Parveen

make these components of melanogenesis dysfunctioned which ultimately lead to pigmentary disorders. Drugs like nonsteroidal anti-inflammatory drugs, antimalarial and tetracycline were found to cause dermatitis followed by pigmentary disorders more often, hyperpigmentary ones [4]. Likewise others including bindi, cheap cosmetics, certain clothes, food allergens *etc.* can also have an impact on skin pigmentation.

There are various dermatoses associated with pigmentation defects that can be congenital or acquired, systemic or skin restricted, temporary or permanent. As these dermatoses have a significant impact on person's quality of life [5], pharmaceutical and cosmetic industries have been continuously searching for solution because their treatment can be disappointing. But it is well said that prevention is better than cure, so in order to make the skin stunning which is free from pigmentary defects, some preventive measures have to be taken care of. Thus, the present chapter is an attempt to enlighten the possible preventive approach of hypo and hyperpigmentation.

2. FORMATION OF MELANIN IN THE SKIN

Pigmentation in vertebrates including mammals is the result of synthesis and distribution of melanin in the skin and hair bulbs. Melanin is produced inside the specialized organelle, melanosome of melanocytes through the complex process of melanogenesis [6, 7]. Melanin plays an essential role in shielding the host from harmful ionizing radiation including UV radiation and in the absorption of free radicals generated within the cytoplasm. Melanin can be of two types: eumelanin and pheomelanin. Eumelanin is the black or brown pigment and pheomelanin is red or yellow [8, 9].

Melanin produces through a series of oxidative reactions involving the amino acid tyrosine in the presence of the enzyme tyrosinase [10]. In the first step, tyrosinase converts tyrosine into dihydroxyphenylalanine (DOPA) and then to DOPA quinone, it is a very critical step as the result of the reaction can proceed spontaneously at a physiological pH. Consequently, DOPA quinone gets converted to dopachrome through autooxidation and then to dihydroxyindole or dihydroxyindole-2-carboxylic acid (DHICA) to form eumelanin. In the presence of cysteine, dopaquinone is converted to cysteinyl DOPA which then produces pheomelanin, a yellow red pigment [11 - 13].

3. PIGMENTARY DISORDERS AT A GLANCE

Any defect affecting the complex process of melanogenesis may result in the onset of pigmentary disorders, which may be either hypopigmentary or hyperpigmentary. The lack or loss of melanin causes hypopigmentation of the skin. These disorders have been the most enigmatic issues since the early days of human civilization. These disorders may be congenital, localized or generalized and may occur as separated or be associated with a wide range of acquired or congenital disorders [14]. Vitiligo, albinism, Vogt-Koyanagi-Harada syndrome, idiopathic guttate hypomelanosis, pityriasis alba are various forms of hypopigmentation [15, 16].

The accumulation of excess of melanin and its distribution causes skin hyperpigmentation. This condition is not considered normal as hyperpigmented macules of variable size have been observed on the exposed areas of the person suffering from hyperpigmentation disorders. Post inflammatory hyper-pigmentation, melasma, ephelide, solar lentigines, purigo pigmentosa, erythema dyschromicum perstans, lichen planus pigmentosus are the diseases involving hyperpigmentation [15 - 18].

4. PREVENTIVE APPROACHES TO SKIN HYPO AND HYPERPIGMENTATION OF SKIN

It has been discussed in the previous chapters that the treatment strategies for skin hypopigmentation and hyperpigmentation do not seem satisfactory so the prevention from these disorders is the best way to go. There are various factors which can directly or indirectly affect the skin pigmentation:

4.1. Drugs and Antibiotics

It has been observed that several drugs consumed by the patients to cure their ailments cause abnormal cutaneous pigmentation. Hyperpigmentation is the most commonly reported cutaneous adverse effects of these drugs. The drugs found to implicate skin pigmentation are non steroidal anti-inflammatory drugs, antimalarial, tetracycline, amiodarone, psychotropic drugs, cytotoxic drugs and metal containing drugs.

4.1.1. Non Steroidal Anti-Inflammatory Drugs

The occurrence of pigmented lesions is associated with non steroidal anti-inflammatory drugs such as salicylates, antipyrine, aminopyrine, dapsone, acetaminophen, oxyphenbutazone, oxicam derivatives *etc*. It has been also reported with many other medications including sulphonamides and phenacetin. The pathogenesis of these drug induced pigmentation is not fully understood but it has been hypothesized that the drug might act as a hapten which binds to the protein linked with melanocytes, the melanocyte consequently becoming the target of a cytotoxic reaction directed toward the offender drugs [19].

4.1.2. Amiodarone

Amiodarone is the anti-arrhythmic and coronary vasodilator which has been known to induce distinctive blue-grey or purple discoloration of the face, nose and ears. Corneal pigmentation is more frequently seen after the treatment with amiodarone but hyperpigmentation of skin appears after 6 months of therapy [20]. The mechanism of induced hyperpigmentation by this drug is still hypothetical but might involve the lipofuscin deposition in dermal histiocytes that contain dense bodies of osmiophilic material. Pigmentation is slow and usually reversible after discontinuation of the drug, but pigmentary lesion may persist for about 1 year [19].

4.1.3. Antimalarial

It has been observed that around 25% of the patients received antimalarial drugs including mepacrine, mefloquine, chloroquine and hydroxychloroquine will develop a bluish grey to dark purple pigmentation [21]. Pigmented lesions appear on anterior side of the leg, nose, cheeks, forehead, ear and oral mucosa. Deeper structures such as ear cartilage, nose cartilage, joint tissues *etc.* are also get affected. Lesions are isolated, oval macules and progressively spread to merge in large lesion. The pathological diagnosis of antimalarial drug induced hyperpigmentation revealed that there is accumulation of melanin and hemosiderin in lower epidermis and dermis. The pigmentation is reversible but the pigmentary lesions disappear after few months [22, 23]. Apart from hyperpigmentation, antimalarial drugs usually chloroquine may also give rise to hypopigmented macules, which involves chiefly the hair or lentigines. Although, these hypopigmented macules disappear within a few months [24].

4.1.4. Tetracycline

Minocycline, an antibiotic of tetracycline group has been reported to induce pigmentary changes. Around 15% of the patients who received minocycline in long duration treatment developed hyperpigmentation [25]. Factors affecting the risk of developing hyperpigmentation include the duration of treatment, daily dosage, presence of previous skin variation related to sun exposure and the associated intake of other pigmentation inducing medications [26].

Minocycline induced pigmentary disorders appear after few months of treatment and have been divided into four clinical patterns (1) Blue black lesions in areas of acne scars or at site of previous skin inflammation; (2) Localized or diffused hyperpigmented lesions from the site of infection for which the antibacterial has been administered; (3) diffuse brown grey hypopigmentation, often called as muddy skin syndrome; (4) Hyperpigmentation of the vermilion portion of the lower lip. The pathological mechanisms of these alterations have not been fully understood but it is assumed that excessive production of melanin occur on sun exposed or inflammatory areas by a direct affect of antibacteria on melanocytes [27 - 29].

4.1.5. Chemotherapeutic Drugs for Cancer Treatment

The cytotoxic drugs used for the treatment of cancer causes skin hyperpigmentation. It affects all parts of teguments including nails, hairs, mucous membrane [30 - 32]. Pigmented lesions can be localized or diffuse. The patho-mechanism is different and largely depends on the type of chemotherapeutic drug. It may involve any of the mechanisms: a toxic affect on melanocytes with stimulation of melanin synthesis; adrenal toxicity which may result in hypersecretion of corticotrophin and melanocyte stimulating hormone; drug-melanin complex formation; post inflammatory hyperpigemntation followed by toxicity of keratinocytes with or without photosensitivity [33]. The pigmentation fades when the cytotoxic drugs induction has stopped. But in rare cases, the lesions are permanent. The cytotoxic drugs which induce hyperpigmentation include cisplatin, hydroxyurea, doxorubicin, idarubicin, bleomycin, docetaxel. Ifosfamide, flurouracil, tegafur, mitoxantrone *etc.* [34 - 45].

4.1.6. Psychotropic Drugs

Phenothiazines and tricyclic antidepressant may induce pigmentation on their long term usage. Chlorpromazine, a phenothiazine is the most frequently used drug which impart violet, purple-grey metallic pigmentation. It affects the mucous membrane but nail beds and exposed areas of the eye also get affected. The pathological examination showed the pigment granules within the macrophages present in the dermis. Ultrastructural studies have revealed that the pigment granules were the complex of the drug and melanin [46, 47]. The other phenothiazines such as trifluoperazine, levomepromazine and thioproperazine have been reported to resolve the problem of hyperpigmentation caused by chlorpromazine [48 - 50].

Tricyclic antidepressant may also be found to induce blue to slate grey hyperpigmentation but much less frequently than chlorpromazine. Desipramine and imipramine are the tricyclic antidepressants which have been reported to induce hyperpiegmentation. Histological examination showed the granules of desipramine and melanin within the macrophages scattered in dermis [51, 52]. Apart from these drugs, there are a large number of chemicals used for several human ailments which may cause skin discoloration. Some of these are clofazimine-used for leprosy; rifampin-used for tuberculosis; zidovidine- used for HIV; hydantoin, phenytoin and barbiturates-anticonvulsants [53 - 58].

Avoidance of such drug induced skin discoloration is not easy because medication of daily usage is more essential than its adverse effects particularly in case of cytotoxic drugs as it is given as life saving treatment. But in other cases, a careful adjustment of the daily doses according to the body weight and age has been done. Another way to avoid drug induced skin discoloration is to decrease sun exposure as much as possible, as it triggers the hyperpigmentation activity of the said drug. In some cases, like with chlorpromazine, it can be replaced by the molecule of the same group without inconvenience.

4.2. Hair Dyes

Para phenylenediamine (PPD) is an amine which has been used as an ingredient in hair dyes. Studies have showed that several hair dyes containing phenylene-diamine cause contact dermatitis followed by pigmentary disorders. The incidence of hypopigmentation due to PPD has been increasing particularly in younger patients [59 - 61].

Henna dye on the other hand is the vegetable hair dye, so it can be used by the people who are sensitized to oxidative dyes. It is the dark green powder, extracted from the leaves of the plant henna, (*Lawsonia inermis*). Temporary skin tattooing using henna has also gained popularity nowadays. For tattooing purpose, certain additives like paraphenylenediamine have been added to henna to make the color of the henna darker. It has been observed that the patients, who have used henna tattooing, developed allergic contact dermatitis with residual hypopigmentation [62, 63]. Recently, Woo *et al.* [64] have showed that the henna dye has affected skin dermatitis followed by dyspigmentation to the Korean patients. Slate grey color dyspigmentation on the lateral side of the face and neck was observed in 8 (72%) patients among the total of 11 patients.

4.3. Cheap Cosmetics

People usually apply cosmetics on their face to look good, which are available as creams, oils, ointments, gels, facewash and soaps. These products contain different constituents which are harmful to the skin and cause pigmentary disorders. The excessive use of these products is due to lack of education, give fast profit for sellers and have low price [65]. Cosmetic tattooing on the other hand also causes severe problems of skin, including discoloration. Nowadays, cosmetic tattooing using micro pigmentation is gaining much popularity. Grey to smoky hyperpigmentation was found in women of 35 years, which is the after effect of permanent lip makeup. Clinical examination diagnosed the multiple pigmented macules as a sequel of cosmetic lip micropigmentation [66]. Similarly, it was reported that Bindi worn on the centre of the foreheads by the women of Indian subcontinent also cause contact depigmentation [67 - 72]. So, it is important to avoid these types of cosmetics and tattoos to protect the skin from having pigmentary disorders.

Certain food also acts as allergen and causes skin dermatitis followed by pigmentary disorders. Some vegetables and fruits when eaten with a specific vegetable or other fruits cause pigmentary lesions on skin. Likewise fish and milk when consumed together causes white spots on skin [73, 74]. Natural allergens like histamine and biogenic amines, excessive sun exposure, certain clothes like nylon and polyesters, post surgical complexes, improper physiotherapy are the various other factors which affect pigmentary change in the patient.

In all the above discussed factors, it is far easier to prevent induced pigmentation from occurring than to treat it. Exposure to sun has been avoided as much as possible because it not only increases the melanin production but also enhances the medication mediated melanin synthesis, which finally leads to skin hyperpigmentation. Protection from sun rays has been done by wearing protective clothes and hats and by applying sun screen of good SPF (sun protection factor). One should discontinue the use of cosmetics and hair dyes which induces abnormal pigmentation. Physiotherapy can be done in a proper way to avoid pigmentary patches on the skin. Likewise people should not eat the food which may cause skin dermatitis and they should avoid the substances which act as allergens on the skin, leading to hypo or hyperpigmentation.

CONCLUSION

The less or excess synthesis of melanin by the melanocytes leads to pigmentary disorders, which can be either hypopigmentary or hyperpigmentary in nature. Although there are various factors which may cause pigmentary disorders but some of them can be controlled so as to prevent the skin from hypo or hyperpigmentation. Certain drugs, antibiotics, improper physiotherapy, hair dyes, cosmetics, food allergens *etc.* may cause pigmentary disorders. It is important to adopt preventive approaches rather to treat them after the onset of the disease as prevention is much easier than to treat the disease. So, avoid or discontinue the use of the things which causes skin dyspigmentation or hyperpigmentation. Physical therapies or post surgical procedures can be done in a proper way.

REFERENCES

[1]　Lin, J.Y.; Fisher, D.E. Melanocyte biology and skin pigmentation. *Nature,* **2007**, *445*(7130), 843-850.
[http://dx.doi.org/10.1038/nature05660] [PMID: 17314970]

[2]　Costin, G.E.; Hearing, V.J. Human skin pigmentation: melanocytes modulate skin color in response to stress. *FASEB J.,* **2007**, *21*(4), 976-994.
[http://dx.doi.org/10.1096/fj.06-6649rev] [PMID: 17242160]

[3]　Park, H.Y.; Kosmadaki, M.; Yaar, M.; Gilchrest, B.A. Cellular mechanisms regulating human melanogenesis. *Cell. Mol. Life Sci.,* **2009**, *66*(9), 1493-1506.
[http://dx.doi.org/10.1007/s00018-009-8703-8] [PMID: 19153661]

[4]　Dereure, O. Drug-induced skin pigmentation. Epidemiology, diagnosis and treatment. *Am. J. Clin. Dermatol.,* **2001**, *2*(4), 253-262.
[http://dx.doi.org/10.2165/00128071-200102040-00006] [PMID: 11705252]

[5]　Ebanks, J.P.; Wickett, R.R.; Boissy, R.E. Mechanisms regulating skin pigmentation: the rise and fall of complexion coloration. *Int. J. Mol. Sci.,* **2009**, *10*(9), 4066-4087.
[http://dx.doi.org/10.3390/ijms10094066] [PMID: 19865532]

[6]　Seiberg, M.; Paine, C.; Sharlow, E.; Andrade-Gordon, P.; Costanzo, M.; Eisinger, M.; Shapiro, S.S. Inhibition of melanosome transfer results in skin lightening. *J. Invest. Dermatol.,* **2000**, *115*(2), 162-167.
[http://dx.doi.org/10.1046/j.1523-1747.2000.00035.x] [PMID: 10951231]

[7]　Schaffer, J.V.; Bolognia, J.L. The melanocortin-1 receptor: red hair and beyond. *Arch. Dermatol.,* **2001**, *137*(11), 1477-1485.
[http://dx.doi.org/10.1001/archderm.137.11.1477] [PMID: 11708951]

[8]　Raper, H.S. The anaerobic oxidases. *Physiol. Rev.,* **1928**, *8*, 245-282.
[http://dx.doi.org/10.1152/physrev.1928.8.2.245]

[9]　Olivares, C.; Jiménez-Cervantes, C.; Lozano, J.A.; Solano, F.; García-Borrón, J.C. The 5,6-dihydroxyindole-2-carboxylic acid (DHICA) oxidase activity of human tyrosinase. *Biochem. J.,* **2001**, *354*(Pt 1), 131-139.
[http://dx.doi.org/10.1042/bj3540131] [PMID: 11171088]

[10]　Shi, Y.L.; Benzie, I.F.F.; Buswell, J.A. Role of tyrosinase in the genoprotective effect of the edible mushroom, *Agaricus bisporus. Life Sci.,* **2002**, *70*(14), 1595-1608.
[http://dx.doi.org/10.1016/S0024-3205(01)01546-6] [PMID: 11991248]

[11]　Kobayashi, T.; Vieira, W.D.; Potterf, B.; Sakai, C.; Imokawa, G.; Hearing, V.J. Modulation of melanogenic protein expression during the switch from eu- to pheomelanogenesis. *J. Cell Sci.,* **1995**, *108*(Pt 6), 2301-2309.
[PMID: 7673350]

[12]　Borges, C.R.; Roberts, J.C.; Wilkins, D.G.; Rollins, D.E. Relationship of melanin degradation products to actual melanin content: application to human hair. *Anal. Biochem.,* **2001**, *290*(1), 116-125.
[http://dx.doi.org/10.1006/abio.2000.4976] [PMID: 11180945]

[13]   Halaban, R.; Patton, R.S.; Cheng, E.; Svedine, S.; Trombetta, E.S.; Wahl, M.L.; Ariyan, S.; Hebert, D.N. Abnormal acidification of melanoma cells induces tyrosinase retention in the early secretory pathway. *J. Biol. Chem.,* **2002**, *277*(17), 14821-14828.
[http://dx.doi.org/10.1074/jbc.M111497200] [PMID: 11812790]

[14]   Dessinioti, C.; Stratigos, A.J.; Rigopoulos, D.; Katsambas, A.D. A review of genetic disorders of hypopigmentation: lessons learned from the biology of melanocytes. *Exp. Dermatol.,* **2009**, *18*(9), 741-749.
[http://dx.doi.org/10.1111/j.1600-0625.2009.00896.x] [PMID: 19555431]

[15]   Plensdorf, S.; Martinez, J. Common pigmentation disorders. *Am. Fam. Physician,* **2009**, *79*(2), 109-116, 109-116.
[PMID: 19178061]

[16]   Fistarol, S.K.; Itin, P.H. Disorders of pigmentation. *J. Dtsch. Dermatol. Ges.,* **2010**, *8*(3), 187-201.
[PMID: 19788584]

[17]   Halder, R.M.; Grimes, P.E.; McLaurin, C.I.; Kress, M.A.; Kenney, J.A., Jr Incidence of common dermatoses in a predominantly black dermatologic practice. *Cutis,* **1983**, *32*(4), 388-390, 390.
[PMID: 6226496]

[18]   Grimes, P.E. Management of hyperpigmentation in darker racial ethnic groups. *Semin. Cutan. Med. Surg.,* **2009**, *28*(2), 77-85.
[http://dx.doi.org/10.1016/j.sder.2009.04.001] [PMID: 19608057]

[19]   Granstein, R.D.; Sober, A.J. Drug- and heavy metal--induced hyperpigmentation. *J. Am. Acad. Dermatol.,* **1981**, *5*(1), 1-18.
[http://dx.doi.org/10.1016/S0190-9622(81)70072-0] [PMID: 6268671]

[20]   Delage, C.; Lagacé, R.; Huard, J. Pseudocyanotic pigmentation of the skin induced by amiodarone: a light and electron microscopic study. *Can. Med. Assoc. J.,* **1975**, *112*(10), 1205-1208.
[PMID: 47784]

[21]   Dubois, E.L. Antimalarials in the management of discoid and systemic lupus erythematosus. *Semin. Arthritis Rheum.,* **1978**, *8*(1), 33-51.
[http://dx.doi.org/10.1016/0049-0172(78)90033-1] [PMID: 358397]

[22]   Koranda, F.C. Antimalarials. *J. Am. Acad. Dermatol.,* **1981**, *4*(6), 650-655.
[http://dx.doi.org/10.1016/S0190-9622(81)70065-3] [PMID: 6165744]

[23]   Bailin, P.L.; Matkaluk, R.M. Cutaneous reactions to rheumatological drugs. *Clin. Rheum. Dis.,* **1982**, *8*(2), 493-516.
[PMID: 6216041]

[24]   Ribrioux, A. [Synthetic antimalarials and skin]. *Ann. Dermatol. Venereol.,* **1990**, *117*(12), 975-990.
[PMID: 2150584]

[25]   McGrae, J.D., Jr; Zelickson, A.S. Skin pigmentation secondary to minocycline therapy. *Arch. Dermatol.,* **1980**, *116*(11), 1262-1265.
[http://dx.doi.org/10.1001/archderm.1980.01640350052013] [PMID: 6449178]

[26]   Simons, J.J.; Morales, A. Minocycline and generalized cutaneous pigmentation. *J. Am. Acad. Dermatol.,* **1980**, *3*(3), 244-247.
[http://dx.doi.org/10.1016/S0190-9622(80)80186-1] [PMID: 6450226]

[27]   Pepine, M.; Flowers, F.P.; Ramos-Caro, F.A. Extensive cutaneous hyperpigmentation caused by minocycline. *J. Am. Acad. Dermatol.,* **1993**, *28*(2 Pt 2), 292-295.
[http://dx.doi.org/10.1016/0190-9622(93)70037-T] [PMID: 8436641]

[28]   Patel, K.; Cheshire, D.; Vance, A. Oral and systemic effects of prolonged minocycline therapy. *Br. Dent. J.,* **1998**, *185*(11-12), 560-562.
[http://dx.doi.org/10.1038/sj.bdj.4809867] [PMID: 9885428]

[29]   Eisen, D.; Hakim, M.D. Minocycline-induced pigmentation. Incidence, prevention and management. *Drug Saf.,* **1998**, *18*(6), 431-440.
[http://dx.doi.org/10.2165/00002018-199818060-00004] [PMID: 9638388]

[30]   Bronner, A.K.; Hood, A.F. Cutaneous complications of chemotherapeutic agents. *J. Am. Acad. Dermatol.,* **1983**, *9*(5), 645-663.
[http://dx.doi.org/10.1016/S0190-9622(83)70177-5] [PMID: 6643764]

[31]   Hendrix, J.D., Jr; Greer, K.E. Cutaneous hyperpigmentation caused by systemic drugs. *Int. J. Dermatol.,* **1992**, *31*(7), 458-466.
[http://dx.doi.org/10.1111/j.1365-4362.1992.tb02689.x] [PMID: 1500233]

[32]   Susser, W.S.; Whitaker-Worth, D.L.; Grant-Kels, J.M. Mucocutaneous reactions to chemotherapy. *J. Am. Acad. Dermatol.,* **1999**, *40*(3), 367-398.
[http://dx.doi.org/10.1016/S0190-9622(99)70488-3] [PMID: 10071309]

[33]   Baselga, E.; Drolet, B.A.; Casper, J.; Esterly, N.B. Chemotherapy-associated supravenous hyperpigmentation. *Dermatology,* **1996**, *192*(4), 384-385.
[http://dx.doi.org/10.1159/000246423] [PMID: 8864385]

[34]   Pratt, C.B.; Shanks, E.C. Letter: Hyperpigmentation of nails from doxorubicin. *JAMA,* **1974**, *228*(4), 460.
[http://dx.doi.org/10.1001/jama.1974.03230290016006] [PMID: 4406195]

[35]   Werner, Y.; Törnberg, B. Cutaneous side effects of bleomycin therapy. *Acta Derm. Venereol.,* **1976**, *56*(2), 155-158.
[PMID: 58526]

[36]   Hrushesky, W.J. Unusual pigmentary changes associated with 5-fluorouracil therapy. *Cutis,* **1980**, *26*(2), 181-182.
[PMID: 7408538]

[37]   Guillet, G.; Guillet, M.H.; de Meaux, H.; Gauthier, Y.; Sureve-Baseille, J.E.; Geniaux, M.; Orreteguy, C. Cutaneous pigmented stripes and bleomycin treatment. *Arch. Dermatol.,* **1986**, *122*(4), 381-382.
[http://dx.doi.org/10.1001/archderm.1986.01660160031013] [PMID: 2420286]

[38]   Kumar, L.; Kochipillai, V. Mitoxantrone induced hyperpigmentation. *N. Z. Med. J.,* **1990**, *103*(883), 55.
[PMID: 2304701]

[39]   Llistosella, E.; Codina, A.; Alvarez, R.; Pujol, R.M.; de Moragas, J.M. Tegafur-induced acral hyperpigmentation. *Cutis,* **1991**, *48*(3), 205-207.
[PMID: 1935249]

[40]   Perlin, E.; Ahlgren, J.D. Pigmentary effects from the protracted infusion of 5-fluorouracil. *Int. J. Dermatol.,* **1991**, *30*(1), 43-44.
[http://dx.doi.org/10.1111/j.1365-4362.1991.tb05878.x] [PMID: 1993564]

[41]   Konohana, A. Blue-gray pigmentation in a patient receiving doxorubicin. *J. Dermatol.,* **1992**, *19*(4), 250-252.
[http://dx.doi.org/10.1111/j.1346-8138.1992.tb03218.x] [PMID: 1318885]

[42]   Gropper, C.A.; Don, P.C.; Sadjadi, M.M. Nail and skin hyperpigmentation associated with hydroxyurea therapy for polycythemia vera. *Int. J. Dermatol.,* **1993**, *32*(10), 731-733.
[http://dx.doi.org/10.1111/j.1365-4362.1993.tb02745.x] [PMID: 8225715]

[43]   Yule, S.M.; Pearson, A.D.; Craft, A.W. Ifosfamide-induced hyperpigmentation. *Cancer,* **1994**, *73*(1), 240-241.
[http://dx.doi.org/10.1002/1097-0142(19940101)73:1<240::AID-CNCR2820730141>3.0.CO;2-6]
[PMID: 8275433]

[44]   Kwong, Y.L. Hydroxyurea-induced nail pigmentation. *J. Am. Acad. Dermatol.,* **1996**, *35*(2 Pt 1), 275-

276.
[http://dx.doi.org/10.1016/S0190-9622(96)90353-9] [PMID: 8708039]

[45]   Borecky, D.J.; Stephenson, J.J.; Keeling, J.H.; Vukelja, S.J. Idarubicin-induced pigmentary changes of the nails. *Cutis,* **1997,** *59*(4), 203-204.
[PMID: 9104543]

[46]   Wolf, M.E.; Richer, S.; Berk, M.A.; Mosnaim, A.D. Cutaneous and ocular changes associated with the use of chlorpromazine. *Int. J. Clin. Pharmacol. Ther. Toxicol.,* **1993,** *31*(8), 365-367.
[PMID: 8225679]

[47]   Mårs, U.; Larsson, B.S. Pheomelanin as a binding site for drugs and chemicals. *Pigment Cell Res.,* **1999,** *12*(4), 266-274.
[http://dx.doi.org/10.1111/j.1600-0749.1999.tb00760.x] [PMID: 10454295]

[48]   Bloom, D.; Krishnan, B.; Thavundayil, J.X.; Lal, S. Resolution of chlorpromazine-induced cutaneous pigmentation following substitution with levomepromazine or other neuroleptics. *Acta Psychiatr. Scand.,* **1993,** *87*(3), 223-224.
[http://dx.doi.org/10.1111/j.1600-0447.1993.tb03360.x] [PMID: 8096668]

[49]   Lal, S.; Bloom, D.; Silver, B.; Desjardins, B.; Krishnan, B.; Thavundayil, J.; Thompson, T. Replacement of chlorpromazine with other neuroleptics: effect on abnormal skin pigmentation and ocular changes. *J. Psychiatry Neurosci.,* **1993,** *18*(4), 173-177.
[PMID: 8104031]

[50]   O'Croinin, F.; Zibin, T. Re: Replacement of chlorpromazine with other neuroleptics: effect on abnormal skin pigmentation and ocular changes. *J. Psychiatry Neurosci.,* **1994,** *19*(3), 226.
[PMID: 8031748]

[51]   Narurkar, V.; Smoller, B.R.; Hu, C.H.; Bauer, E.A. Desipramine-induced blue-gray photosensitive pigmentation. *Arch. Dermatol.,* **1993,** *129*(4), 474-476.
[http://dx.doi.org/10.1001/archderm.1993.01680250086012] [PMID: 8466219]

[52]   Sicari, M.C.; Lebwohl, M.; Baral, J.; Wexler, P.; Gordon, R.E.; Phelps, R.G. Photoinduced dermal pigmentation in patients taking tricyclic antidepressants: histology, electron microscopy, and energy dispersive spectroscopy. *J. Am. Acad. Dermatol.,* **1999,** *40*(2 Pt 2), 290-293.
[http://dx.doi.org/10.1016/S0190-9622(99)70467-6] [PMID: 10025850]

[53]   Karat, A.B.A.; Jeevaratnam, A.; Karat, S.; Rao, P.S. Controlled clinical trial of clofazimine in untreated lepromatous leprosy. *BMJ,* **1971,** *4*(5786), 514-516.
[http://dx.doi.org/10.1136/bmj.4.5786.514] [PMID: 4942741]

[54]   Holdiness, M.R. A review of the Redman syndrome and rifampicin overdosage. *Med. Toxicol.,* **1989,** *4*(6), 444-451.
[http://dx.doi.org/10.1007/BF03259925] [PMID: 2689837]

[55]   Gallais, V.; Lacour, J.P.; Perrin, C.; Ghanem, G.; Bodokh, I.; Ortonne, J.P. Acral hyperpigmented macules and longitudinal melanonychia in AIDS patients. *Br. J. Dermatol.,* **1992,** *126*(4), 387-391.
[http://dx.doi.org/10.1111/j.1365-2133.1992.tb00686.x] [PMID: 1315150]

[56]   Gallais, V.; Lacour, J.P.; Ortonne, J.P. [Cutaneous pigmentation disorders in human immunodeficiency virus infection]. *Ann. Dermatol. Venereol.,* **1992,** *119*(6-7), 471-478.
[PMID: 1280021]

[57]   Hammer, C.J. Melasma induced by oral contraceptive drugs. *Northwest Med.,* **1968,** *67*(3), 251-254.
[PMID: 5649712]

[58]   Baker, H. Adverse cutaneous reaction to oral contraceptives. *Br. J. Dermatol.,* **1969,** *81*(12), 946-949.
[http://dx.doi.org/10.1111/j.1365-2133.1969.tb15983.x] [PMID: 4312248]

[59]   McFadden, J.P.; Yeo, L.; White, J.L. Clinical and experimental aspects of allergic contact dermatitis to para-phenylenediamine. *Clin. Dermatol.,* **2011,** *29*(3), 316-324.
[http://dx.doi.org/10.1016/j.clindermatol.2010.11.011] [PMID: 21496741]

[60]   Handa, S.; Mahajan, R.; De, D. Contact dermatitis to hair dye: an update. *Indian J. Dermatol. Venereol. Leprol.*, **2012**, *78*(5), 583-590.
[http://dx.doi.org/10.4103/0378-6323.100556] [PMID: 22960813]

[61]   Encabo Durán, B.; Romero-Pérez, D.; Silvestre Salvador, J.F. Allergic Contact Dermatitis Due to Paraphenylenediamine: An Update. *Actas Dermosifiliogr.*, **2018**, *109*(7), 602-609.
[http://dx.doi.org/10.1016/j.adengl.2018.06.017] [PMID: 29496197]

[62]   van Zuuren, E.J.; Lavrijsen, A.P. [Allergic reactions and hypopigmentation due to temporary tattooing with henna]. *Ned. Tijdschr. Geneeskd.*, **2002**, *146*(28), 1332-1335.
[PMID: 12148222]

[63]   Jovanovic, D.L.; Slavkovic-Jovanovic, M.R. Allergic contact dermatitis from temporary henna tattoo. *J. Dermatol.*, **2009**, *36*(1), 63-65.
[http://dx.doi.org/10.1111/j.1346-8138.2008.00588.x] [PMID: 19207440]

[64]   Woo, Y.R.; Kim, J.S.; Lim, J.H.; Choi, J.Y.; Kim, M.; Yu, D.S.; Park, Y.M.; Park, H.J. Acquired diffuse slate-grey facial dyspigmentation due to henna: an unrecognized cause of pigment contact dermatitis in Korean patients. *Eur. J. Dermatol.*, **2018**, *28*(5), 644-648.
[PMID: 30530434]

[65]   Jaccob, A.A.; Yaqoub, A.A.; Rahmani, M.A. Impact of abuse of topical corticosteroids and counterfeit cosmetic products for the face: prospective demographic study in Basrah City, Iraq. *Curr. Drug Saf.*, **2019**, *15*(1), 25-31.
[http://dx.doi.org/10.2174/1574886314666191001100357] [PMID: 31573892]

[66]   Abtahi-Naeini, B.; Shahmoradi, Z.; Hadian, M.; Niknami, E.; Saffaei, A. Multiple pigmented macules as a sequel of cosmetic lip micro-pigmentation: New clinical presentation of tattoo reactions. *Niger. Postgrad. Med. J.*, **2019**, *26*(4), 244-246.
[http://dx.doi.org/10.4103/npmj.npmj_88_19] [PMID: 31621666]

[67]   Bajaj, A.K.; Govil, D.C.; Bajaj, S. Bindi depigmentation. *Arch. Dermatol.*, **1983**, *119*(8), 629.
[http://dx.doi.org/10.1001/archderm.1983.01650320003003] [PMID: 6870313]

[68]   Pandhi, R.K.; Kumar, A.S. Contact leukoderma due to 'Bindi' and footwear. *Dermatologica,* **1985**, *170*(5), 260-262.
[http://dx.doi.org/10.1159/000249545] [PMID: 4007222]

[69]   Kumar, A.S.; Pandhi, R.K.; Bhutani, L.K. Bindi dermatoses. *Int. J. Dermatol.*, **1986**, *25*(7), 434-435.
[http://dx.doi.org/10.1111/j.1365-4362.1986.tb03447.x] [PMID: 3771039]

[70]   Bajaj, A.K.; Gupta, S.C.; Chatterjee, A.K. Contact depigmentation from free para-tertiary-butylphenol in bindi adhesive. *Contact Dermat.*, **1990**, *22*(2), 99-102.
[http://dx.doi.org/10.1111/j.1600-0536.1990.tb01525.x] [PMID: 2323209]

[71]   Mathur, A.K.; Srivastava, A.K.; Singh, A.; Gupta, B.N. Contact depigmentation by adhesive material of bindi. *Contact Dermat.*, **1991**, *24*(4), 310-311.
[http://dx.doi.org/10.1111/j.1600-0536.1991.tb01736.x] [PMID: 1868725]

[72]   Bose, S.K. Is Bindi-induced depigmentation common in patients predisposed to vitiligo? *J. Dermatol.*, **1994**, *21*(5), 370-371.
[http://dx.doi.org/10.1111/j.1346-8138.1994.tb01756.x] [PMID: 8051327]

[73]   Sternberg, T.H.; Bierman, S.M. Unique syndromes involving the skin induced by drugs, food additives, and environmental contaminants. *Arch. Dermatol.*, **1963**, *88*, 779-788.
[http://dx.doi.org/10.1001/archderm.1963.01590240103018] [PMID: 14071450]

[74]   Watemberg, N.; Urkin, Y.; Witztum, A. Phytophotodermatitis due to figs. *Cutis,* **1991**, *48*(2), 151-152.
[PMID: 1935241]

SUBJECT INDEX